The History of Medicine in Twelve Objects

The History of Medicine in Twelve Objects

DR CAROL COOPER

Aurum

First published in hardback in 2024 by Aurum,
an imprint of Quarto
One Triptych Place,
London, SE1 9SH
United Kingdom
www.Quarto.com/Aurum

A catalogue record for this book is
available from the British Library.

ISBN: 978-0-7112-9462-2
E-book ISBN: 978-0-7112-9464-6
Audiobook ISBN: 978-0-7112-9618-3

2 4 6 8 10 9 7 5 3 1

Cover design by Anna Morrison
Typeset in Bembo Infant MT by seagulls.net
Printed and bound by CPI Group (UK) Ltd, Croydon, CR0 4YY

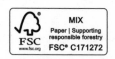

Contents

Introduction *p1*

1. The Trephine: Like a Hole in the Head *p9*

2. The Bone Saw: Cutting-Edge Surgery *p31*

3. The Mask and Personal Protection *p49*

4. The Microscope and the Hidden World
of Germs *p71*

5. The Stethoscope: Listening to the Patient *p93*

6. The Ether Inhaler and the Conquest of Pain *p117*

7. The Hypodermic Needle and Syringe: at the Sharp
End of Treatment *p139*

8. Obstetric Forceps: Modern Methods for Birthing
Babies *p163*

9. The X-Ray Machine: Making the
Body Transparent *p187*

10. The ECT Machine and Shocking Approaches
to Mental Illness *p215*

11. The Prosthetic Hip: A Triumph of Orthopaedics *p237*

12. The Heart-Lung Machine: How the
Impossible Became Possible *p257*

Timeline *p283*
Acknowledgements *p291*
Picture credits *p292*
Index *p293*

This book is dedicated to the memory of
George Ashley Cooper and Elizabeth Edwards Cooper.

Introduction

As archaeology confirms, ill health has been with us since the beginning of time, along with a desperate need to treat it. In the beginning, remedies were purely experimental, as brave practitioners and even braver patients embarked on treatments on a kill-or-cure basis.

Understanding what causes disease has mostly lagged behind empirical treatments. Scientific knowledge often arrived in the wake of a bold procedure, whether it succeeded or not. Along the way, setbacks have followed breakthroughs, as medics and the sick encountered wrong turns and dead ends. All of us today owe so much to the ingenuity of those who came up with new tools to deal with baffling symptoms, especially when those instruments led to further study and the accumulation of proper evidence. And so the history of medicine has rolled out, albeit in fits and starts, taking a great many casualties along the way. Most of them were patients, but not all.

Just twelve objects? How can it be possible, you may wonder, to retell the development of modern medicine in just a dozen devices. It is a tiny number in relation to the range of paraphernalia deployed today. All the same, this varied collection covers most medical specialities. The objects range in size, too. Some items could sit in the palm of your hand while others need the best part of a room.

No list of instruments can be definitive. The choice here reflects my own professional practice and teaching, as well as my bias, I'm sure. Each chapter takes one object and shows its place in the history of healthcare, which includes the subsequent development of more advanced tools and techniques. The CT scanner, for instance, doesn't get its own chapter, because it developed from the X-ray machine. And sometimes the invention of an object has enabled advances in fields other than the one for which it was first intended.

Each object speaks. It comes from a certain era. It may be typical of a particular culture. A device tells us about the practice of medicine at the time, and about its inventors. Yes, an instrument can have several. It's unusual for a groundbreaking idea to come from the brainwave of a lone genius. American physician and poet Oliver Wendell Holmes (1809–94) put it well: 'Genius comes in clusters, and rarely shines as a single star.' You may think of Thomas Edison (1847–1931) as the inventor of the light bulb, but it was Humphry Davy (1778–1829) who set it all off with his work on electric arc lighting, Americans William Sawyer (c.1850–83) and Albon Man (1826–1905) who patented the incandescent light bulb, and Joseph Swan (1828–1914) who obtained the patent in England. Edison himself acknowledged that he did not invent the light bulb out of nothing. He did, however, create a carbonized bamboo fibre that made an excellent filament, and he went on to make a name for himself with other developments, including motion pictures.

Sometimes innovations take shape at the workbench of more than one person or team at roughly the same time, as if the concept hung in dust motes in the air, waiting to be caught. Synchronicity can lead to disputes over priority and patents. The victor is usually the one with the best publicity. If there's a celebrity endorsement, you're home and dry, as in the case of John Snow (1813–58) who gave Queen Victoria chloroform when she laboured with her eighth child.

Many early medical objects were barely more than lethal weapons. It seems a miracle that any patients survived their procedures, especially at a time when those wielding the devices had little idea of what they were doing. Imaginative practitioners sometimes developed fanciful theories for what ailed their patient and the way in which their treatment had worked. However, until science entered the scene, these explanations were no better than a bedtime story. No wonder the French writer Voltaire (1694–1778) is said to have described the art of medicine as 'entertaining the patient while nature effects the cure'.

As witty as Voltaire's dictum was, it was only true in the days when plants, poultices, and prayer held sway over science. After the Industrial Revolution, medicine and technology became partners, and treatments grew more rational. Even so, a new way of doing things was not always immediately accepted, and its proponent was often ridiculed.

Patients were not necessarily willing participants. Consent is a modern concept. In times past, it rarely applied to sick humans, and it has never applied to animals. Medical advances bear the indelible stain of vivisection. As any biologist should realize, animals are sentient beings, yet they are treated for the most part as experimental material, or just another tool. It's contradictory and illogical to justify the use of testing on animals on the grounds that they are so similar to humans, yet at the same time deny that they too can feel pain and have emotions.

I decided to keep the hard science simple in this book. 'Decided' may not be quite the right word, since I've long forgotten the meagre physics I ever understood. Apologies to those who might have preferred more details. You won't find a single equation here. I've concentrated more on why and how the inventions came about. There will be familiar names, among them Joseph Lister, Louis Pasteur, Marie Curie, and Hippocrates, alongside many other people whose lives I hope you will enjoy getting to know. Apologies, too, if your favourite tool or trailblazer isn't here. I could have included many more names, but the book might have read like a telephone directory.

The trailblazers were for the most part men. It's only recently that women have breached the doors of medicine and make their mark. Until the nineteenth century (and even well beyond), men generally believed that women were ill-equipped to be doctors on all fronts – physical, emotional, and intellectual. They mustered specious arguments for their opinion. Women were not rational enough. Their brain was inferior. Evolution had passed them by. And so on. Psychiatrist Henry Maudsley (1835–1918) even believed that women could develop either brains or ovaries, but not both.

In 1872, the *Lancet* declared that women doctors were 'contradictory to nature'. By then, the English suffragist Elizabeth Garrett Anderson (1836–1917) had already qualified as a physician and surgeon. She had many obstacles to negotiate. The Royal College of Surgeons of England stipulated a long apprenticeship, at least three years' study, courses in dissection, and an exam. Women were barred from all of these. Garrett circumvented the hurdles in 1865 by gaining a licence from the Society of Apothecaries instead, making her the first woman to qualify in Britain. The Society of Apothecaries immediately changed its charter to exclude other women, so that others had even more trouble following in her footsteps.

It should be no surprise that women make good doctors. Over 200 years ago, surgeon Astley Cooper (1768–1841) addressed students at St Thomas' Hospital in London and summed up the most desirable attributes of a surgeon as the eye of an eagle, the heart of a lion, and the hand of a lady. This was probably based on an old English maxim, so it was not new even in 1815, but ever since then it has been strongly linked with Cooper.

But then new ways of doing things, like new instruments, take time to be accepted. As economist John Maynard Keynes (1883–1946) said, 'The difficulty lies not so much in developing new ideas as in escaping from old ones.'

I hope you enjoy reading about ideas and objects old and new, and about the people who brought them about.

Carol Cooper

The
History of
Medicine
in Twelve
Objects

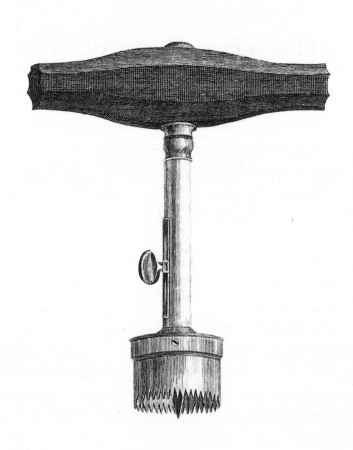

1

The Trephine:
Like a Hole in the Head

A trephine is a borer or small saw used to make holes in the skull. Technically, a trephine is a device with three ends (from the Latin *tres fines*) that is held by two of the ends with the third one making a hole, while a trepan (from the Greek *trypanon*/τρυπανον) literally means a drill or bore. A purist will say the two objects are different, but trephines and trepans basically do the same job. The question is, why would anyone want a hole in the head in the first place?

The history of trepanning – which you could also call trepanation or trephining – goes back to the Mesolithic era. Humans have had holes made in their skulls before either recorded history or metal tools. With archaeological evidence going back to 10,000 BCE or so, trepanning is sometimes called the oldest human surgical procedure, though both circumcision and limb amputation have the edge as they go back even further. Still, it's safe to say that trepanation was the first neurosurgical procedure performed on humans.

It was surprisingly widespread. Trepanned skulls have been found in Mesoamerica, South America, Africa, Asia, and Europe. At that time, populations were less mobile than today. How trepanation evolved in so many disparate places and in different cultures around the globe is as puzzling as why it was done. What may also be surprising is that many patients survived the procedure, which we can deduce from the skull regrowth seen in many skeletons. The operation could have had a ritual function, at least in some African cultures and pre-Columbian Mesoamerica. Later, though, the Egyptians, Greeks, and Romans definitely used it as a medical treatment.

Early instruments used for trepanation were sharpened stones. Mark II trepans were wooden tools. Later, metal trepans came into use. The holes they made varied in shape and size. Some were round or oval, like the burr holes that neurosurgeons drill into the skull today, while other openings were far more ragged.

Trepanation became a serious scientific procedure with Hippocrates of Kos (c.460–c.370 BCE). Hippocrates classified skull fractures and gave instructions on trepanation, including warnings on the dangers of venturing into the brain. In his writings, he advises the operator to stop clear of the dura mater, the outermost of the three layers of meninges or membranes around the brain. This made excellent sense if you wanted the patient to live.

While Hippocrates didn't get everything right, he used evidence and was a rational man who avoided superstition. His book *On Injuries of the Head*, written around 400 BCE (though possibly not all by him), is the earliest manual of operative neurosurgery and full of sage advice. In it, he details the management for each type of skull trauma (contusions, linear fractures, depressed fractures, and so on). Interestingly, he advises against trepanation for depressed skull fractures, which is the opposite of what's done today. Hippocrates liked to use a serrated trepan, checking the depth of the hole repeatedly with a sound as he went along. Experience taught him that damaging the meninges could lead to infection, brain abscess, and death. Seizures could also result from penetrating the meninges. These occurred on the opposite side of the body from the injury, which was a significant observation because it showed that certain nerve pathways must cross the midline on their way from the brain to the limbs.

Six centuries after Hippocrates, neurosurgery made another leap forward. The physician Galen (129–216 CE) came from Pergamon, now in Turkey but at that time a sizeable Greek city. After studying at the Aesculapion of Pergamon, a sanctuary to the god of healing, he gained expertise at the Alexandria school of medicine. Returning to Pergamon, he was appointed physician to the gladiators. Their injuries were frequent and often severe, so there was plenty of hands-on experience. Galen also began using trepanation to treat depressed skull fractures.

During Galen's time, trepanation became more sophisticated, as did the instruments he developed. Some had guards on them to reduce the risk of injury. Typically, the patient sat up for the procedure. There wasn't much lighting, so this gave a better view. It also helped blood drain away, which was vital as the scalp has many blood vessels.

Substances were sometimes applied to the edges of a scalp incision to stem blood flow, as well as act as some sort of antiseptic. Most of these products were just chemical irritants and worked, if they did at all, by causing local inflammation. Galen tried mixtures of vinegar, honey, and salt, as well as various unguents that contained plant extracts, pigeon blood, black coral, and a miscellany of other ingredients that must have seemed a good idea at the time.

In his studies, Galen described anatomical entities in the brain such as the corpus callosum, the ventricles, the pineal, the pituitary, and the cranial nerves. He also encouraged doctors to practise their operating on animals first.

Galen produced reams of original work in all fields of medicine, some four million words in all, although a fire nine years before his death destroyed much of it. Undaunted, he continued researching and writing. His ideas persisted until sometime during the sixteenth century. His success also earned him accolades, including his appointment as physician to Commodus (161–92 CE), son of Marcus Aurelius (121–80 CE).

Around the globe, different populations must have trepanned for different reasons. In South America, bone discs the same size as the skull holes have occasionally been unearthed. Some of these have small holes drilled through them, as though they were meant to be worn as amulets. A few of the discs must have been gouged out post-mortem, but, on the whole, trepanation was done during life, and the extent of bone formation proves that the patients lived quite a while after the procedure.

The eighteenth century was a particularly busy time for trepanning, and European doctors were fond of the practice. They used trepanation to treat concussion and brain inflammation. In the nineteenth century, trepanation was widely used during the American Civil War (1861–5) to deal with head wounds. At one point, Cornish miners demanded that their skulls be trepanned if they had a head injury, regardless of whether there was a fracture.

In Peru and other parts of South America, trepanation was most popular between the fourteenth and sixteenth centuries. Anaesthesia may have been provided in the form of coca leaves, which acted as a local painkiller. A significant finding in the history of trepanation goes back to 1865 in Cuzco, Peru. American Ephraim George Squier (1821–88), archaeologist and diplomat, was at one point the guest of a Señora Zentino, who was known as a collector of art and antiquities. Zentino had a number of skulls on display in her personal collection, one of which had a square hole in it. When Squier admired it, the generous Zentino gave it to him as a present.

The skull, dating from 1400–1530 CE, was from an Inca burial ground, and the hashtag-shaped hole on its right side was clearly made on purpose, probably with a semicircular instrument called a burin. Squier noted that the individual must have survived the operation for some time.

The skull was presented at a meeting of the New York Academy of Medicine. The learned audience reacted with scepticism. Racism and xenophobia may have reared their heads, too. How could someone from a primitive and foreign culture have carried out such a procedure when in the United States the survival rate from similar surgery was at the time under 10 per cent?

Squier then took his Peruvian skull to Europe's foremost authority on the comparative study of skulls. Frenchman Paul Broca (1824–80) was an anthropologist as well as professor of clinical surgery at the University of Paris – more of that career later. His special interest was skulls from different races and cultures around the world. Having examined the Squier skull (as most call it), Broca and his colleagues agreed that the hole in the skull was due to trepanation and that the patient had survived for a while. In 1876, Broca presented his findings to the Société d'anthropologie de Paris. As in New York, astonishment reigned. This type of surgery was surely too demanding and too refined to have been the handiwork of Peruvian Indians. Archaeological evidence forced Europeans to realize that primitive societies were perhaps not all that primitive after all. However, the importance of trepanation in terms of modern medicine is in its lasting contribution to anatomy, neurology, and neurosurgery.

∞

Experience with people who'd had accidents contributed to the concept of localization of brain function. In one celebrated case, brain trauma led to radically changed behaviour.

It came to be known as the 'American Crowbar Case.' In 1848, Phineas P. Gage, a twenty-five-year-old construction worker on the Rutland and Burlington Railroad, was severely injured while excavating rock to build a railway line in Vermont. He was tamping explosive powder into a drill hole, but a premature detonation sent his tamping iron – a long bar over a 1 m (3¼ ft) long and weighing 6 kg (13¼ lb) – sailing through his head. The metal rod went through his left cheek and the left frontal lobe of his brain, then out through the vault of his skull on the right.

He remained conscious, though he continued to bleed. The vision in his left eye had gone, and his face drooped because the facial nerve on that side was damaged. When he developed an infection, he was deemed to be close to death. A coffin was even made for him. But the care of his doctor, John Martyn Harlow (1819–1907), helped him survive, albeit with immediate mental and behavioural changes that everyone noticed. Once energetic, friendly, and hard-working, Gage became irresponsible, stubborn, foul-mouthed, and generally uninhibited. The only thing he was motivated to do was carry that tamping iron everywhere he went.

Impressed by his patient's survival of the ordeal, Harlow followed Gage in his travels across North and South America. After Gage died of epileptic seizures in California in 1860, the doctor retrieved the skull and the tamping iron. Harlow left both items to Harvard Medical School's anatomical museum, and later most of his own money to charity.

The case became well known among doctors after Harlow wrote it up in a medical journal. Later, Gage's personality changes were recognized as part of frontal lobe syndrome. The frontal lobe, especially the part called the orbito-frontal cortex, deals with emotion and affect, as well as coordinating such things as planning, motivation, decision-making, and social behaviour. There is no one single task for this part of the brain. Some other parts, however, are more specialized.

Paul Broca was a celebrated surgeon and neurologist, as well as an anthropologist. In 1861, he had a patient by the name of Louis Victor Leborgne. He was of normal intelligence but had developed an inability to speak, apart from saying the syllable *tan*. For some reason, Leborgne developed gangrene and other serious problems, and died while under Broca's care. Post-mortem showed a lesion in the posterior region of the left frontal lobe. Within just a few years, Broca found eight more patients with similar lesions, prompting him to declare, '*Nous parlons avec "hémisphere gauche"!*' (We speak with the left hemisphere). He was right, or at least he was in the case of 95 per cent of right-handed people and 75 per cent of left-handers. Specifically, we speak with a part of the left side of the brain now called Broca's area, and patients like Louis Leborgne are said to have 'Broca's aphasia'. Over a dozen other anatomical regions also bear Broca's name, as medical students soon discover.

Broca also wrote many articles on the pathology of bones and joints, aneurysms, craniometry, and physical anthropology, inventing measuring instruments that are still in use. He clashed with the Catholic Church, which wanted to stop the teaching of anthropology. Broca was only fifty-six when he died. He was survived by his wife and two sons, both of whom became distinguished professors of medicine.

In 1874, the German physician Carl Wernicke (1848–1905) studied a group of patients who, in contrast to Broca's, could speak but not understand. He pinpointed a lesion in the posterior part of the temporal lobe. Unsurprisingly, the condition is often called 'Wernicke's aphasia'. Wernicke also gave his name to a number of other medical conditions.

The brain, once a box full of mystery, was gradually revealing some of its workings. John Hughlings Jackson (1835–1911), a physician from York, can be thought of as the founder of modern neurology. He was made a Fellow of the Royal Society, and his ideas on the organization of the brain endure today. He concluded that diseases of the nervous system might not necessarily involve the nerves themselves, but could be disorders of blood vessels, for example. Knowing the exact organ was, in his view, vital to a correct diagnosis. Seizures were Hughlings Jackson's main area of interest. He described one type of fit that begins on one side of the body and is now called Jacksonian epilepsy, and another type called temporal lobe epilepsy (TLE). TLE refers to partial seizures that commonly include feelings of déjà-vu, fear, panic, nausea, and sometimes hallucinations of smells.

Neurologist Hughlings Jackson and the author Henry James (1843–1916) had many friends and associates in common. In James's gothic novella *The Turn of the Screw* (1898), the governess is prone to seeing things that unsettle her deeply. The 'turn' of the title almost certainly refers to the governess's funny turns. James describes these in detail, and many doctors are convinced that her diagnosis was TLE. James is believed to have obtained his medical knowledge directly from Hughlings Jackson.

In a twist of fate, Hughlings Jackson's wife died of a blood clot on the brain, her condition having been complicated by Jacksonian epilepsy.

The practical upshot of this growing mountain of knowledge of the brain was soon to follow in the form of brain surgery, if only a patient and his doctor proved brave enough. That patient was a twenty-five-year-old farmer from Dumfries called Mr Henderson. Nobody seems to know what his given name was. For three years, the muscles on the left side of his face had twitched uncontrollably. The spasms worsened. He developed seizures during which he lost consciousness. By the time he was admitted to London's Hospital for Epilepsy and Paralysis in 1884, he was unable to move his left arm and had developed unbearable headaches.

His neurologist there was Alexander Hughes Bennett (1848–1901). After examining Henderson, he concluded that the trouble was a small but growing tumour in the fissure of Rolando (the central sulcus of the brain), not far from his right ear. Initially Henderson was treated with drugs, but even generous doses of morphine did nothing for his pain and distress. His days were miserable and at night his screams kept the whole ward awake. The only option was to remove the tumour. It had never been tried before, but Henderson was desperate and willing to risk his life.

The brave surgeon was thirty-five-year-old Rickman J. Godlee (1849–1925), a nephew of Joseph Lister (1827–1912) and well acquainted with the principles and practice of antisepsis. Godlee was a highly skilled surgeon, albeit not actually a neurosurgeon, since this speciality didn't exist at the time. Apart from Hughes Bennett, several other notable neurologists were in the operating theatre with Godlee and his patient, as were several assistants. The two-hour operation employed chloroform as anaesthetic, while assistants sprayed carbolic. It was a team effort to localize and remove the tumour, which turned out to be a glioma the size of a walnut.

Early results were remarkably good. Henderson's headaches and seizures vanished. Unfortunately, infection set in despite antisepsis. Henderson developed meningitis and lived only four weeks after this landmark surgery. In the words of the old saw, the operation was successful, but the patient died.

As an interesting aside, the neurologist Hughes Bennett himself developed a mysterious neurological illness that caused him great pain and loss of mobility. Nobody seems quite sure of the diagnosis, but it forced him to retire at the age of just forty-five. He died eight years later.

Also present in the operating room with Godlee and his patient Henderson was one David Ferrier (1843–1928), a Scottish neurologist and psychologist who published *The Functions of the Brain* (1876), a book detailing thousands of experiments on live animals, many of them monkeys, cats, and dogs. Ferrier used a host of techniques including electrical stimulation. In 1881, he became the first scientist to be prosecuted under the Cruelty to Animals Act (1876), but he was acquitted.

Godlee's operation drew a great deal of attention. For one thing, it was the first time that a surgeon had been able to remove a tumour from within the human brain, so it represented the dawn of modern brain surgery. For another, it fuelled fierce debate on the research that had made it possible. Victorian England saw the vocal emergence of sentiment against vivisection. Questions included whether findings from animal research could safely be extrapolated to humans. In any case, could the cruelty of animal experimentation be morally justified, even when it led to useful advances? Was vivisection always for the public good, or was it more often in the cause of personal advancement for its practitioners? Did it make those engaged in it callous and dehumanized? These were unanswered at the time, and are still hot questions that polarize opinion today.

∞

The first neurosurgeon of the twentieth century was the American Harvey Cushing (1869–1939). Cushing was the youngest of ten children and became the first surgeon to work exclusively in neurosurgery, as well as the world-leading teacher of neurosurgeons of his time. Today he is best remembered for describing Cushing's syndrome, caused by overproduction of steroids from the cortex of the adrenal glands. If pushed to say what kind of doctor Cushing had been, most medical students would probably plump for 'physician' or 'endocrinologist'. In fact, Cushing's greatest achievements probably took place in the operating theatre, and he may have saved many more lives with his contributions to neurosurgery than with his description of Cushing's syndrome.

When he was an intern in 1895, patients often bled to death on the table during brain surgery. Cushing changed that with a strict surgical regime. He operated aseptically and controlled bleeding slowly and fastidiously. In his able hands, mortality dropped from 50 to 10 per cent. He introduced X-rays to help localize brain tumours. He also busied himself with research, much of it using electrical stimulation of the cortex.

A perfectionist, Cushing was not an easy man. His sharp tongue would reduce nurses and junior doctors to tears. He disapproved of a long list of things, among them jazz, telephones, movies, stylish clothes, women in medicine, and women smoking. Cushing was himself a heavy smoker but, when faced with leg amputation for gangrene of the toes, he gave up cigarettes instead and promptly improved. Decades before research had proven smoking was harmful, he became a passionate advocate for quitting. After he died of a heart attack, post-mortem revealed a cyst in the third ventricle of the brain. It had caused no symptoms.

History should also celebrate Wilder Graves Penfield (1891–1976) and his work in the early twentieth century. Penfield was an American-Canadian neurosurgeon. A handsome man, he started out as an all-American boy: a good college student, athlete, and class president. He had applied to Princeton University because his mother had chosen it for him. At the time, Rhodes Scholarships were awarded on a state-by-state basis, and New Jersey is a small state. He duly became a Rhodes scholar. He studied at Oxford and elsewhere, learned from world-famous doctors including Harvey Cushing, travelled widely, served in the First World War, got injured, completed his PhD at Johns Hopkins, and practised for several years at NewYork-Presbyterian Hospital.

Most medics know him for mapping the sensory areas of different parts of the body in the cerebral cortex – the so-called cortical homunculus. A homunculus literally means 'little man' in Latin. A cortical homunculus is a distorted map (or a three-dimensional figure) of the human body, based on the area of the brain devoted to each part of the body. The figure looks distorted with oversized lips, hands, feet, and genitals, because these areas have more sensory neurones than other parts of the body. The motor homunculus is similar to the sensory homunculus. Although most homunculi are specifically little men, finally there are now female homunculi.

Penfield should also be remembered for his humanity. One of his first patients in New York was a boy with a brain tumour. As Penfield had to explain to the parents, he could do nothing to save the boy's life because the tumour was too deep to remove. But, he added, 'I may be wrong. Doctors are wrong sometimes, you know.' From then on, his abiding principle was never to remove all hope.

In Canada, he established the Montreal Neurological Institute and continued his research. His so-called 'Montreal procedure' for epilepsy dates from 1952. It enables surgeons to destroy the brain cells where seizures originate. Under local anaesthetic, it's possible to stimulate parts of the brain with electricity and ask the patient to describe the sensations triggered. This allows doctors to identify and eliminate areas of the brain that produce seizures (or the aura that can precede a seizure, such as smelling burnt toast). Thanks to the procedure, Penfield also discovered a lot more, including which parts of the brain produce certain thoughts and how memories are stored.

Penfield spent his last fifteen or so years writing articles, medical biographies, and novels. Some of his writings speculated on the nature of human consciousness and the mysteries of the soul.

∝

Almost all the advances described so far relate more to brain function than to its structure. In fact, anatomists as far back as antiquity had studied the brain. The early Greek scientist and philosopher Alcmaeon of Croton, born around 510 BCE, suggested that the brain rather than the heart ruled the body, which was a controversial view at the time. To study the brain and vision, he set about dissecting brains and eyes.

Two other important Greek anatomists were Herophilus (335–280 BCE) and Erasistratus (c.304–c.250 BCE) who both worked in Alexandria and founded a school of anatomy there. They were busy dissectors of the human brain, and many of their ideas persist today. These two were the first Greek physicians to undertake thorough dissections of human cadavers. Until then, there had been repugnance at the concept as well as religious and moral taboos. But Herophilus and Erasistratus were fortunate in their timing. They had royal patronage and an abundance of recently executed criminals. This was the era of the Ptolemies, the Greek rulers who were keen to establish Alexandria as a dazzling hub for scientific endeavour and literary achievement – they also encouraged the building of the library of Alexandria. At the time, Alexandria was highly cosmopolitan, and remained so until the 1960s. After Herophilus and Erasistratus, anatomy almost disappeared, until, some four centuries later, Galen (129–216 CE) came onto the scene. He was interested in anatomy, of course, but Roman law had prohibited the dissection of human cadavers since about 150 BCE.

There were few anatomical strides made during the so-called Dark Ages (the fifth to fourteenth centuries), and no wonder. Christianity had it that the soul was of prime importance and the body was too trivial to be worth studying. Dissection of human cadavers was forbidden, and scientists had only previous works to rely on.

Then came the Renaissance, and with it Vesalius (1514–64), whom most consider to be the outstanding ana-tomist of his age. He relied on earlier work, notably Galen's (some of which was inaccurate), but he also carried out his own meticulous dissections. Vesalius had a wonderful eye for detail and his drawings were exceptional. His elegant artwork isn't just stunning. It clearly shows structures of the brain, like the caudate nucleus, the thalamus, the stria terminalis, the fornix, the hippocampus, the superior and middle cerebral peduncles, and more. This is particularly remarkable as Vesalius had only a few cadavers to work on and he had to move fast. The tissues of the brain decom-pose quickly, and several of the corpses that came his way also had to be dissected at speed for legal reasons.

The work of Vesalius set the stage for the continu-ing development of the science of anatomy. As attitudes towards human dissection began to mellow and modern information added to the knowledge in Galen's texts, the descriptions of the gross anatomy of the brain became quite detailed. Still, nobody yet knew what might lie within all these structures.

With the invention of the microscope in the seven-teenth century (see Chapter 4), the microanatomy of the brain could also be studied. It became accepted that the tissues of the body were made up of cells. However, brain tissue was hard to study. Under the lens, it sometimes looked like a homogeneous grey mush. It became possible to make sense of the microscopic appear-ance of the brain only after Italian biologist Camillo Golgi

(1843–1926) developed improved cell staining techniques in the 1870s.

Together with Spanish neurologist Santiago Ramon y Cajal (1851–1934), Golgi won the Nobel Prize in 1906 for studies of the structure of the nervous system. Their opinions differed at first. Ramon y Cajal believed that the nervous system was made up of individual cells, while Golgi maintained that it was a protoplasmic syncytium – a single complex cell with several nuclei. But, when Golgi's staining procedures were used, Ramon y Cajal showed that the nervous system was, as he'd maintained all along, composed of discrete units, or neurones (also known as neurons).

❦

Neurosurgery has travelled a long way since the trepanations of 10,000 BCE. Today, it makes use of microscopy, endoscopy, CT and MRI scanning, endovascular techniques (for instance, for carotid endarterectomy), laser instrumentation, and robotics.

The control of bleeding has moved on since the days of pigeon blood and black coral. Cushing pioneered electrocautery, but there are now also a plethora of different haemostatic agents that are useful where cautery can't be used. There are sealants, like fibrin glue and polymers. There are also gelatine sponges, collagens, oxidized cellulose, and polysaccharide spheres that can all act on contact with the site of bleeding to encourage platelets to clump together and form a clot. Then there are agents that actively take part in the biochemical cascade of changes that produce a clot. They're more expensive that the first type, but also more effective, even in patients with deficient platelets. A further type of agent incorporates these last two.

Anaesthetics have progressed vastly, too, especially when you consider that the time-honoured way to operate on the skull was while the patient was fully conscious. These days, awake craniotomy is still a useful option. A conscious patient can help the surgeon operate with greater precision, for instance by saying what sensations he experiences. He can also speak up if the surgeon triggers the aura of his seizures. If surgery is on the dominant hemisphere, the patient can read or talk during the operation, to avoid losing an area essential to speech. Awake should not mean distressed. There are now anaesthetics, often two or more drugs used together, that will ease pain, sedate without interfering with patient cooperation, and produce amnesia so that the whole experience is a smooth one.

If you think the age-old practice of trepanation is no longer with us, you may be surprised to learn that it still has fans today. A few people claim that the procedure, done as a DIY project with a power drill, can improve blood flow to the brain and bring physical and spiritual benefits. The theory put forward for this bizarre belief is that, when our skull bones harden in infancy and fuse along the sutures, blood flow is compromised and can thus lead to a higher risk of neurodegenerative disease.

The author Lobsang Rampa went even further with his enthusiasm for openings in the head. In his 1956 book *The Third Eye*, he described how a small hole made in the middle of his forehead aroused 'the third eye' and bestowed supernatural powers. Allegedly written by a Tibetan monk, the book became a bestseller. The author who called himself Lobsang Rampa was later discovered to be one Cyril Henry Hoskin (1910–81), a plumber from Devon who had only been to Tibet in his imagination.

Perhaps needless to say, there is no scientific basis for any of these fanciful claims for trepanation. Blood reaches the brain via the carotid and vertebral arteries, not by diffusion through the sutures. The risks of DIY trepanation are high and include infection and brain damage. In fact, were you to compile a roll call of procedures that shouldn't be tried at home, this one deserves to be very near the top of the list.

At one point, John Lennon was a fan of trepanation. It's on record that he tried to persuade fellow Beatle Paul McCartney to have the procedure. In the end, good sense prevailed and neither of them opted to go under a trepan.

You may like to know that nowadays there are other more conventional surgical trephines, many of them small devices with a serrated blade and used for procedures such as corneal grafting, bone marrow biopsy, and frontal sinus drainage.

A kind of trepanation can also come in handy if you drop something heavy on your toe, or if your finger is crushed in a door. An accumulation of blood under the nail can be painful and may even lift the nail off. Therefore, if you have a large or painful subungual haematoma, you may be offered trephination with a sterile needle to drain the blood. The nail itself will feel nothing of the procedure, unlike the skulls of those patients of old.

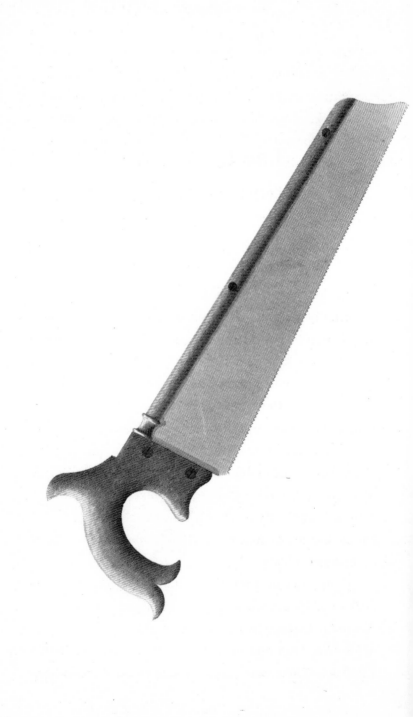

2

The Bone Saw:
Cutting-Edge Surgery

If necessity is the mother of invention, the bone saw is the offspring of limb amputation. As a deliberate procedure, amputation began a long time ago. The earliest saws or blades were thought to date from around 10,000–8,000 BCE, and at least some patients survived their agonizing and bloody ordeal. But recent findings suggest the operation may go back even further. One skeleton from Indonesian Borneo is that of a child whose lower leg was amputated in about 31,000 BCE. Subsequent bone growth shows that he managed to live a good few years after that. There were no metal saws at the time, so how it was done is uncertain, but the fact it was done at all suggests some understanding of the human body.

Bone saws in a form we might recognize today go back to 3,500 BCE when they were fashioned from copper. As metal extraction processes evolved, tougher blades made from iron and steel came into use around 1,400–1,200 BCE. These were strong enough to cut through bone

31

in a straight line. Ruins from Pharaonic times (about 3,000 BCE–323 CE) depict amputations, as do amphoras and mosaics from Ancient Greece and Rome.

Before anaesthesia and antisepsis, amputation was excruciating and hazardous. Battlefield injuries were the principal rationale for amputation, and were the main reason why the operation and its instruments evolved. As Hippocrates is said to have written, 'He who wishes to be a surgeon should go to war.'

He was right in that wars led to many improvements in surgery. But they were not the only driver. Violence was common in civilian life, and for millennia life was nasty, brutish, and short. Justice could be harsh too. Doctors of today sometimes think patients and their families are overly demanding, but the Ancient Babylonian legal text, the Code of Hammurabi (c.900–1750 BCE), states that a physician could expect a hand to be amputated if the patient failed to improve under their care. Aside from trauma and punishment, grounds for amputation included severe burns, chronic infection, gangrene, vascular disease, frostbite, and tumours. There were few other treatments for these conditions. Amputation may have been the last resort, but in many cases it was the only resort.

During the Renaissance, surgery and instruments progressed apace, led by barber-surgeons. The role of barber-surgeon has monastic origins from about 1,000 CE. Each monastery had to hire or train a barber to keep the tonsure of Catholic monks in trim. On the side, a barber-surgeon would also perform a little minor surgery like teeth-pulling and procedures such as the application of leeches.

For centuries, qualified physicians considered manual work beneath them, so they rarely carried out operations. In time, two types of practitioner evolved, those with practical know-how and those who worked in universities and treated the wealthy. The latter did not sully their hands, especially by dealing with the wounded.

It was barber-surgeons that generally treated soldiers in and after battle. The most illustrious of them all was French barber-surgeon Ambroise Paré (*c*.1510–90). He was born into a modest family in Laval, a town roughly halfway between Paris and Brest, and came to be known as one of the Fathers of Surgery. Although his formal education was minimal, he became apprenticed to a barber-surgeon and managed to train for three years at the renowned Hôtel-Dieu in Paris.

The major wars during his lifetime were the long Italian Wars (1495–1559) and the Wars of Religion (1562–98) which were a series of bloody civil conflicts between Protestants and Catholics. Paré became an innovator in military medicine, bringing in new treatments for wounds and for firearms injuries. His work largely consisted of amputations done at speed, for which a saw was essential. Other tools were useful too, like bullet extractors, bone scrapers, knives to cut away the other structures, and suture needles to close the wound. Paré introduced several instruments, such as artery forceps to control bleeding.

Instead of cauterizing arteries, he favoured tying them off, a technique first used by Galen many centuries earlier to stop haemorrhage.

Amputation was done in one circular cut, and it had to be done swiftly. Although germs had not yet been discovered, it was understood that the longer an operation lasted, the more likely the patient was to die. Even more crucial from a practical point of view, the only painkillers at the time were opium, mandrake, alcohol, and henbane, which is related to deadly nightshade. Sometimes, the pain was so severe that patients fainted. If they didn't, they were inclined to scream and leap off the table. To prevent this, anyone who happened to be available, including the surgeon's family, would be volunteered to pin them down.

Paré served as barber-surgeon under the French monarchs Henri II, François II, Charles IX, and Henri III, gaining valuable experience both in peacetime and in war. Celebrated as he was, a good patient outcome was far from certain, and the Almighty was often invoked to help. After he'd treated a captain in the Piémont campaign of 1537–8, Paré wrote: '*Je le pansay et Dieu le guérit*' (I bandaged him and God healed him). This quote is carved into the monument to him in his home town of Laval.

Said to have been intelligent, ambitious, and vain, Paré was also a thoughtful surgeon and a devout Christian – although it was never quite clear whether he was Protestant or Catholic. He gathered evidence and he listened to his patients. Paré first described phantom limb pain, in other words the perception of pain or discomfort in a limb that is no longer there. This type of pain is common after amputation and occurs in some 50–80 per cent of limb amputees. Unlike pain in the stump, which gradually improves as the wound heals, phantom limb pain does not get better on its own. Paré suspected it was due to damage of nerve fibres or even changes in the brain, which is more or less what the experts still believe today.

Alongside his contributions to amputation techniques, Paré also championed a gentler art of surgery. After going under the saw, gunshot patients had their fresh wounds treated with a solution of boiling oil. Other practitioners had long believed it to be a good way to detoxify the wound, but it often caused great pain and swelling. Paré was still in his twenties when a shortage of oil led him to experiment with something less irritant. He concocted a balm of egg yolk, rose oil, and turpentine, and amputees did find it a lot more acceptable. At the time, it was something of an eye-opener that a surgeon would even think of reducing the pain of treatment.

During his long life, Paré also devised trusses for hernias, dealt with nasal afflictions, reimplanted teeth, and fashioned limb prostheses. He even made artificial eyes from enamelled gold, silver, porcelain, and glass.

Even more astonishingly, Paré only used treatments and procedures he had personally observed to be useful. Barber-surgeons of the time did not publish, or even get their knowledge from books. Their teaching was mostly aural. But Paré wrote extensively on surgery and other medical topics, weaving in the evidence he gathered as his experience grew. He didn't know any Latin so he wrote in conversational French. This made his work far more accessible to other barber-surgeons than it would have been in the more traditional Latin. He even illustrated his work, which was another novelty. Soon his writings were translated into German, English, and Dutch, thereby reaching a huge audience. Empiricism spread.

A large part of Paré's legacy was the role he played in raising the standards for training barber-surgeons. The College of St Côme, once so snooty towards barber-surgeons, realized Paré's value. The brothers of the college therefore waived the usual requirement of a Latin exam and welcomed him as a master surgeon in 1554. After the siege of Rouen, Paré went on to even greater heights when he was appointed premier surgeon to the king, Charles IX.

∝∾

The design of bone saws evolved and styles changed. Amputation blades generally curved downwards in the eighteenth century. Over time, these became straighter in order to facilitate amputations in which the surgeon made a flap to cover the bony stump. At the end of the eighteenth century, tenon saws displaced bow saws in Britain, and later they did so in America, though not in continental Europe.

Saw handles also changed. For a long time they were wooden, but from the nineteenth century handles were entirely metal. Nickel plating arrived on the scene in the 1890s and made the blade and the handle harder and less likely to corrode, an important property when they began to be routinely boiled and disinfected.

They changed in weight too. Bow or frame saws were heavy in the seventeenth century, but became gradually lighter and less bulky. Specialized instruments were created, like the metacarpal bow-frame saw for hand amputation. It looked like a modern-day hacksaw.

The French continued to make major advances in trauma surgery, thanks in large part to the Napoleonic Wars (1803–15) that followed on from the French Revolution. One big name of the period is Dominique Jean Larrey (1766–1842), who was chief surgeon to the army and went on every one of Napoleon's campaigns. He was lauded, fêted, and befriended by the emperor. Among his innovations was the *ambulance volante* or flying ambulance. The ambulance did not actually fly. It was a light two-wheeled vehicle pulled by two horses, and it meant that casualties could be retrieved from the battlefield before they bled to death.

Inevitably, amputation was the most frequent operation during conflict. Larrey performed an extraordinary number himself, some of them with a narrow linear saw that he introduced. Instruments to control haemorrhage also came in, but surgery was still painful and hazardous. The more audacious the operation, the greater the risk. Larrey is said to have undertaken the first amputation through the hip joint, a monumental undertaking for both doctor and patient. He carried out this particular operation seven times. His first six patients perished.

This was still before effective anaesthesia, so speed was of the essence, whatever the procedure. In nineteenth-century England, none came much faster than Astley Paston Cooper (1768–1841) of Guy's Hospital. In 1824, he took little more than twenty minutes to amputate a leg through the hip joint, a procedure that had not been done since Larrey and still remains a highly demanding surgery today. Cooper's patient lived.

As a youth, Cooper had been a rebel and a practical joker who often played truant. He grew up to become a surgeon held in high regard, then and now, a man deemed the greatest English operator of his time. He was appointed President of the Royal College of Surgeons twice, in 1827 and 1836. He was also a popular teacher who brought his lessons to life by passing body parts taken from dissection around the lecture theatre. In middle age, he was debonair and mixed with the elite. Although Cooper had no royal appointment, King George IV summoned him to remove an infected cyst from his head. Reluctantly, Cooper operated. Luckily, the surgery went well, and it gained him a baronetcy.

As a lecturer in anatomy at Surgeons' Hall, his work involved publicly dissecting bodies recently removed from the scaffold. It was often hard to find corpses for dissection because, under the Murder Act of 1752, only the bodies of executed murderers could be used. With the flourishing of medical science and the drop in executions, other means for supplying bodies evolved. Grave robbers (also known as resurrectionists or body snatchers) became active. Then there was an Edinburgh duo who went a little further than that. William Burke and William Hare murdered to supply bodies. They were arrested in 1828 and the case caused public revulsion about the whole issue. Something had to be done.

A Select Committee was set up to investigate how bodies should be sourced for anatomy students, and Cooper's testimony helped sway the committee. His some-what high-handed opinion is recorded as: 'The law does not prevent our obtaining the body of an individual if we think proper; for there is no person, let his situation in life be what it may, whom, if I were disposed to dissect, I could not obtain.' Despite dissent from many, the Anatomy Act was passed in 1832. It allowed surgeons to acquire any unclaimed dead bodies, and the legislation remained in place until the Anatomy Act of 1984.

Cooper's name lives on today. Search the textbooks and you may come across Cooper's fascia, Cooper's pubic ligament, Cooper's stripes, Cooper's breast ligaments, Cooper's testis, Cooper's disease, Cooper's hernia, and so on. Rather easier to find is a large statue of him in St Paul's Cathedral, London, holding a thick tome.

A generation after him, the luminous Scottish surgeon Robert Liston (1797–1847) left Astley Cooper's operat-ing speed in the shade. To enable faster amputations, Liston invented a double-edged knife made from high-quality steel with a razor-sharp blade that was usually 15–20 cm (6–8 in) long. He would insert this long knife into the middle of the thigh, parallel to the bone, then withdraw it outwards, slicing the soft tissues as the blade emerged. The Liston knife, as it came to be known, was actually strong enough to slice through bone, but a saw with a serrated blade was still generally used for cutting bone itself. The Liston became the standard amputation knife, as well as a favourite tool of Jack the Ripper (dates and identity unknown).

Liston also invented forceps with a built-in lock that kept the tips together to stop arterial bleeding. His amputation technique was to create a flap of skin and tissue that could be folded over the cut end of the bone to complete the operation, avoiding the usual problems that accompanied a simple circular cut.

Unlike most surgeons of the day who worked in filthy aprons covered in blood, Liston would put on a clean apron for each operation. He was also one of the few to wash his hands before surgery. This was well before microorganisms were discovered, so perhaps he had some innate sense of tidiness and order. All the same, Liston did not appear to find anything wrong with holding his knife between this teeth now and again during surgery.

As an operator, Liston was astonishingly fast. From start to finish, an above-knee amputation might take him between thirty seconds and two-and-a-half minutes. Visiting surgeons crowded into his operating theatre to admire the great man at work. With theatrical flair, the virtuoso surgeon drew himself up to his full height and urged his audience to keep an eye on their pocket-watches. 'Time me, gentlemen,' he exhorted. 'Time me.'

He was the first professor of clinical surgery at University College Hospital, where he gained a reputation for being the fastest knife in the West End. And his results were excellent, with only one patient in ten succumbing from surgery. At nearby hospitals, the death rate was one in four. His swiftness and precision were awe-inspiring, until the day he lopped off a patient's testicles along with the leg that he was amputating.

Liston is also rumoured to have performed the only operation that had a 300 per cent mortality. During the procedure, he hacked so hastily that he took off one of his assistant's fingers in addition to the patient's leg. In the same fell swoop, he also managed to tear through a visiting professor's coat. Believing he'd been stabbed, the professor lost consciousness and never recovered. The patient died of a wound infection, and the assistant perished of a gangrenous hand. Only Liston survived, if one can believe the tale.

Liston was a fearless doctor who operated on cases where all his colleagues had given up hope. Perhaps surprisingly, he believed that a patient's emotions were important, and he did his bit to allay their fears where he could. They grew a lot less apprehensive with the advent of anaesthesia. Liston is known for the first public operation under ether in Europe, which he performed in 1846. His patient was one Frederick Churchill, a thirty-six-year-old butler from Harley Street with chronic osteomyelitis of the tibia, for which there was no other remedy. The amputation took just twenty-five seconds. Afterwards, Churchill is said to have asked when his op was going to get started.

Liston died at the age of fifty-three from an aortic aneurysm that ruptured as the result of a sailing accident. His main legacy is the impact he made on surgical techniques such as amputation flaps, locking artery forceps, and, of course, the Liston knife. But that may not be all. His high standards, his commanding manner, and his flair for showmanship seem to have become the template for many surgeons since then. He is buried in London's Highgate Cemetery.

While the Liston knife lived on, other amputation instruments changed considerably in style between 1840 and 1860. Cutler Joseph-Frédéric-Benoît Charrière (1803–76) was behind many of the refinements. Swiss by birth, he worked in Paris from the tender age of thirteen and learned to craft instruments from newer materials such as nickel silver and stainless steel (as well as rubber, which he used to manufacture catheters). The Charrière bone saw looks like an upmarket hacksaw and is strong enough to cut through thigh bone. It is still in use today. Charrière became a French citizen at the age of forty, and was inducted into the Légion d'honneur in 1851. He died in Paris when he was seventy-three.

~⤫~

Bone saws developed further during the American Civil War. There are few niceties in wartime, and there were even fewer than usual in this conflict, which was the first war to take place during an industrial age. War brings novel methods of maiming and killing fellow men, and battlefield trauma becomes more complex and more demanding to treat. This hastens surgical innovation, but somehow the destruction of war always keeps a step or two ahead.

In the American Civil War, the standout challenge came from the Minié or Minie ball (pronounced *minnie*). The Minie ball was a kind of hollow-based lead bullet for muzzle-loading muskets. Dating from 1847, it was extensively used in the Civil War by both sides, and busy factories ensured supplies never ran short. Just one person could cast 3,000 Minie balls an hour.

The Minie ball was the brainchild of French military inventor and instructor Claude-Étienne Minié (1804–79). Weighing less than 30 g (1 oz), a Minie ball could send limbs flying and cause far worse injuries than earlier musket balls. That's because the bullet flattened out on impact, leading to further damage to the tissues.

Amputations were especially common since limb-saving treatments for injuries such as gaping wounds and compound fractures weren't always feasible in the field, or even at all after a Minie ball had struck. Various bone saws were used. One of them was a chain saw that allowed the surgeon to reach behind a bone without cutting everything else in sight. This was useful when just a portion of a badly fractured bone could be removed, although inevitably it left that limb much shorter than its opposite number.

The signature instrument of the Civil War, however, was an all-metal tenon saw, most often called the Satterlee bone saw. It was named after Richard Sherwood Satterlee (1798–1880), a medical officer in the US Army, although it was neither designed by him nor even specified by him when he was at the Medical Purveyor's Office in New York City, overseeing the purchase of surgical instruments. The saw was initially marketed in 1872 by manufacturer George Tiemann and Co. (founded in 1826). Some five years later, its description changed to 'Satterlee's capital saw' to reflect its extensive use in the war.

With its pistol-grip handle, the Satterlee saw became the quintessential American bone saw and, in many ways, it still is. It was the standard amputation saw during the First and Second World Wars. Although other saws, mostly motorized, are now used in modern civilian settings, this saw is still being manufactured for use in remote areas and for inclusion in the medical kits for combat hospitals and humanitarian organizations. When a power saw lets a surgeon down, the Satterlee can finish the job.

Leonardo Gigli (1863–1908) pioneered a different type of bone saw altogether. He was an Italian surgeon and obstetrician who cut through the pelvic bone to widen a woman's pelvis for the relief of obstructed labour. The procedure was called lateral pubiotomy, or Gigli's operation. He carried this out with his Gigli saw, a device made of sharp, flexible cable that vaguely echoed the chain saw used in the American Civil War. Pubiotomy has fallen from favour, but Gigli saws are still used today where precision and control are vital: for instance, when opening the skull like a clam shell once burr holes have been made.

More complex procedures have led to the development of new bone saws. In the late nineteenth century, power saws came in. They were initially operated by foot. By 1895, however, the innovative French surgeon Eugène-Louis Doyen (1859–1916) harnessed electricity to boost the power of the saw. He also introduced electrocautery and the Doyen retractor, still used today for pelvic surgery.

Others continued to perfect the power-saw. These days, power tools are the norm for cutting bone, whether it's for amputation or for splitting the sternum to operate on the heart. American orthopaedic surgeon and inventor Homer Hartman Stryker (1894–1980) patented the oscillating saw in 1947. He also brought in micro-reciprocating saws in the late 1960s. These small instruments mimic the back-and-forth action of hand-sawing but are, of course, much faster and more precise. The more efficient the saw, the more bone dust it produces. Stryker developed blades with a channel near the teeth to reduce bone chips building up on the blade or showers of bone fragments dispersing into the operating theatre.

Bone saws also produce unwanted noise and heat. It is wise to avoid generating too much heat because bone adjacent to the cut can undergo necrosis (death of body tissue) if the temperature rises to 47°C (117°F) for one minute, or even just 43°C (109°F) for an hour. Fortunately, laser tools can also be used to cut bone. A laser produces a focused light beam that does increase the temperature of tissues in its path, but doesn't cause friction side effects as mechanical saws do, so laser cutting gives off less heat and can be more precise into the bargain.

Since 1985, when they were first used for prostate biopsies and for some neurosurgical procedures, robotics have played an increasing role in surgery. Bones and joints, with their hard landmarks, are especially amenable to robot-controlled operations. There are several types of robotics. In the so-called active system, the robot is almost autonomous in its ability to cut bone or carry out other actions, as well as to make decisions based on sensors that respond to the operative environment. Active systems need the least direct human input while operating, but, of course, a huge amount of detailed planning is essential pre-op. In a semi-active system, the surgeon operates alongside the robot. Again, meticulous planning is a must. The surgeon uses the robot as a tool for carrying out the operation, with the robotic system giving feedback. This works as a safety feature to ensure that cutting goes exactly as needed in terms of speed and direction. The robot can halt the process if cutting happens to deviate from the plan. Passive robotic systems, on the other hand, function as a kind of map for the operator. They use software and sensors to show where to position the cutting tool. Apart from that, the surgeon carries out the procedure in the time-honoured way. This kind of system is proving its worth in resecting bone tumours, among other uses.

One of the great advantages of robotics in orthopaedic surgery is that these systems can reproduce predictable and consistent angles and locations for the surgeon to cut. This is especially relevant to joint replacement (see Chapter 11, page 248). Another boon is that, unlike a human operator, the robot never gets tired or needs a good night's sleep. In robotic surgery, the surgeon may not have to be in the same hospital or even the same country as the patient. Telemedicine means that surgeons can collaborate to operate on a patient, as long as they agree with one another.

There is a significant cost to robotics, and it's primarily financial. The initial outlay on equipment is high, and surgeons also need extra training to use it, which is another expense. No system is foolproof and there can be operating glitches. If the technology fails for any reason, the procedure may have to be completed in the traditional way. One of the arguments against robotics, or at least against over-reliance on it, is that surgeons can become deskilled in manual operating, and that may only come to light in an emergency, when it's most needed.

For now, Gigli saws are still used for some procedures, while the Satterlee saw and the Liston knife also endure. Barber-surgeons may no longer be with us, but reminders of them live on. Patients in the British Isles are sometimes bemused to find that surgeons don't go by the title of Doctor. As soon as a surgeon acquires a qualification from the Royal College of Surgeons, they leave the title Doctor behind. This tradition harks back to the time of the barber-surgeons who were not medically qualified. Rest assured that today's surgeons are indeed properly certified, and they no longer have a sideline in haircuts.

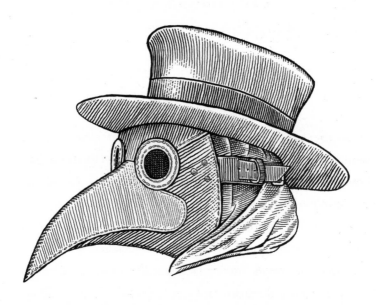

3

The Mask and
Personal Protection

Since the Covid-19 pandemic, almost everyone in the world has grown familiar with surgical face masks. They have become a symbol of our time, as the *New York Times* wrote in early 2020.

While the profusion of discarded masks in the street may be unique to recent years, the history of protective face gear stretches back around two millennia, to an era when nobody suspected the existence of viruses or bacteria, let alone their capacity to cause disease and death. In Roman times, Pliny the Elder (23–79 CE), philosopher and sometime handyman, constructed a mask from animal bladder, but the aim was to avoid breathing noxious mercury dust while he crushed the mineral cinnabar. Leonardo da Vinci (1452–1519) used a wet cloth over his face to protect himself from chemical toxins. That too was for his own well-being. During the Yuan dynasty in thirteenth-century China, on the other hand, servants waiting on the emperor and his court covered their mouths

and noses with silk fabric to stop their breath from taint-
ing the meals they served. Early on, then, there was the
understanding that face coverings could protect either the
wearer or others.

Come the Black Death in the early fourteenth century
and face gear came into its own. Today we know that
bacteria called *Yersinia pestis* caused the Black Death or
plague. Back then, it was blamed on miasma, a belief that
goes back to Hippocrates. Miasma refers to poisonous air
or a blight, often foul-smelling. Some attributed the plague
epidemic to spoiled air from the East, a notion that has
the same xenophobic overtones as referring to Covid-19
as 'the China virus'.

The Black Death swept across the globe in pandem-
ics, each of which killed millions. It devastated Europe
for centuries and left few countries unscathed. In Britain,
about a third of the population is believed to have died. In
Venice, multiple eruptions of the plague ravaged the city
between 1348 and 1528. The symptoms were fearsome:
high fever, strange rashes, suppurating buboes (enlarged
lymph nodes) in the groin, armpit, and neck, a cough, and
blood-stained phlegm, or rapidly fatal sepsis – all depending on the clinical form of the disease. The complete
absence of a cure added to the terror.

When the plague hit Paris in 1619, doctors could do
little for it apart from protect themselves while they tended
to their patients. French physician Charles de Lorme
(*c.*1584–1678) is credited with pioneering the plague doctor
outfit. The most striking element of the ensemble was the

headpiece and mask, with its waxed hood, glass eyepieces, and a long beak-like structure with nostrils. The beak was designed to contain a mixture of herbs like garlic and rue, and spices such as clove and cinnamon, the aim being to purify the air and protect the doctor from contracting the deadly infection. The choice of herbs and spices wasn't based on evidence, but it was doubtless more wholesome than the stink of putrefaction and death.

Docteur de la Peste's get-up also included a top hat, heavy boots, waxed trousers, a long stick for examining patients without getting too close, thick goat-skin gloves just in case, and over it all a long black cloak impregnated with waxes and oils to repel body fluids. The wearer was unrecognizable in this costume, but their appearance at the door must have been all too ominous. Other doctors soon adopted the clever invention, and de Lorme's reputation grew. He became a celebrity in the French court and around Europe. The City of Venice even conferred on him the status of nobleman. It probably did no harm that his father, Jean de Lorme, had been a notable physician who had also looked after French royals. At the age of twenty-six, de Lorme *fils* became primary physician to Henri IV, and then to two of his successors, Louis XIII and Louis XIV.

This was not yet the age of science. De Lorme had a penchant for prescribing unproven remedies, including antimony, a toxic metal he regarded as a sovereign cure for just about anything, especially when added to wine. As with his father, Charles de Lorme had his detractors. Many must have envied his fame. Overall, though, he was clever and charming. He pioneered his protective equipment and remedies, while on the side he would regale patients with lively anecdotes and stories. History remembers him as one of the most famous French doctors.

If your thoughts now turn to another Frenchman, it's worth noting that Louis Pasteur wasn't a clinical doctor. However, two centuries after de Lorme, it was indeed Pasteur who may have done more than anyone else to develop the mask. A microbiologist and chemist, Pasteur (1822–95) described germs as the source of infections (see Chapter 4, page 76). It became clear that patients had to be protected.

In Breslau, surgeon Johann Mikulicz-Radecki worked out how. Mikulicz (1850–1905) had a bacteriologist colleague Carl Flügge (1847–1923), who had recently shown that even normal conversation could disperse bacteria in respiratory droplets. This resonated with Mikulicz, who was already keen on sterile cloth gloves. In 1897, Flügge's findings prompted him to create a face mask made of a single piece of gauze tied with two strings. 'We breathed through it as easily as a lady wearing a veil in the streets,' Mikulicz wrote that same year. Another assistant added to the design with a two-layered mouth protection made of gauze to prevent dribble reaching the patient, which must have been a useful refinement.

Nonetheless, face coverings for surgeons were not immediately popular, a phrase that applies to many if not most medical advances. Until 1910, uptake was patchy but mask use gradually spread as more evidence of microbes emerged. Photos taken of surgical teams in the US and Europe suggest that by 1923 over two-thirds of surgeons wore a mask.

During epidemics, face masks again found uses outside hospitals. In the Manchurian plague, a young Chinese doctor recommended masks to protect both medics and the population. Born in Malaysia, Wu Lien-teh (1879–1960) was the first Chinese student to graduate in medicine from Cambridge, and the first to have his work published in the *Lancet*. His greatest achievement, however, came in 1910–11. Apart from identifying the first case of the Manchurian plague, he urged people to wear masks made of gauze and cotton. That, and his other public health measures, brought the outbreak under control. His influence continued after the plague. Sensitive and erudite, he understood that medicine in China would need to incorporate modern advances alongside traditional healing. Masks again played an important part in the influenza pandemic of 1918–19 and are credited with preventing the spread of infection.

Over time, the device evolved. Paper began to edge out cloth in the 1930s. Soon after, synthetic materials became popular, and the shape of masks changed too. But, as it turned out, sterilization damaged synthetic fabrics. The early 1960s therefore ushered in the era of single-use synthetic masks.

In 1972, the US approved the first single-use N95 respir-ator mask. The rating N95 means that it blocks around 95 per cent of particles that measure 0.3 microns or more, which includes many viruses. The material may look nothing special, but it makes use of electrostatic charge. This gives it the power to trap small particles more effectively than uncharged fabrics. The American technology company 3M developed the N95 thanks to a remarkable design consultant they hired. Sara Little Turnbull (1917–2015) was one of the country's first industrial designers. Born Sara Finkelstein, her adult height was just under 1.5 m (5 ft) so she was nicknamed Little Sara before she eventually adopted Sara Little as her professional name. After success as a child actor, a textile designer, a magazine editor, and a marketing consultant, among other roles, Turnbull turned her hand to working with 3M on a new non-woven fabric. In the 1950s, she devised a number of uses for it, including a moulded bra cup and a medical mask. The N95 mask that eventually resulted has the same basic shape as the bra cup. Unlike the bra, it has a bendable nose clip and is disposable. N95 use grew with the Covid-19 pandemic. Although more expensive than the common types of disposable mask, it was, and still is, easy to buy in shops.

❦

There are situations where a mask alone may protect the patient from infection but is not enough to protect the wearer. Medical visors and face shields, either disposable or reusable, can help form a barrier to particles and body fluids. Specific eye protection was also part of the PPE (personal protective equipment) armamentarium during the Covid-19 pandemic. Its use had become widespread in the 1980s with HIV. Contrary to some surgeons' beliefs, good-quality eye protection doesn't interfere with vision, and it's especially valuable for doctors who may get splashed with body fluid.

Like much clinical paraphernalia, masks are more than medical devices. While a surgical mask only weighs some 5 g (⅙ oz), it is heavy with significance. To many people, masks imply an acceptance of modern medicine and a readiness to protect others, even when it is a little inconvenient. During the Covid-19 pandemic, several public figures declared mask-wearing to be an act of civic duty. To others, they signify government interference and erosion of personal liberty. Those that rejected the value of masks during the pandemic showed their scepticism of medicine and perhaps a rejection of authority in general. So, this rectangle of fabric smaller than a handkerchief not only filters out germs. It also represents beliefs about science and society. Culture has a lot to do with attitudes to masks. In the US, some hold that being obliged to wear a mask is unconstitutional. In Japan, however, masked rail commuters were a common sight long before Covid-19, especially in Tokyo during winter.

For a mask to function well, it needs to fit snugly over both nose and mouth, and that applies just as much to surgeons as the general public. If glasses steam up, it usually means the mask fits badly across the nose. Masks do slip sometimes, but the nose shouldn't poke out over the top. Wearing a mask like a sling for the chin isn't going to do much, either, except make the wearer look ridiculous. Yet that's often what people do when they get uncomfortable.

Some people lower their mask because, they claim, they're unable to breathe with it on. Most of us can, if we're hale and hearty. Nonetheless, prolonged mask-wearing can have consequences, including a rise in carbon dioxide in the blood, a drop in oxygen saturation, and an increase in heart rate and respiratory rate. A less healthy circulation may not be able to compensate for this and in some people, such as children, adolescents, and pregnant women, a rise in carbon dioxide might cause problems. Wearing a mask may trigger headaches, acne, and other facial lesions, as well as panic attacks in those prone to them. A few people describe dizziness, drowsiness, exhaustion, or a combination of these. This set of symptoms has been reported in numerous medical journals and sometimes described as Mask-Induced Exhaustion Syndrome (MIES). At the moment, the medical jury is still out as to its significance. But in the meantime it makes sense not to apply a blanket ruling on masks, or at least not for extended periods of wear.

Speech interpretation often relies on visual clues, so does covering the face hinder communication? Anecdotal evidence suggests that a mask may interfere with understanding. However, studies so far fail to show much impact for either standard-hearing people or those with impaired hearing. In healthcare situations, ambient noise from a dental drill or a floor polisher is probably a more important factor.

A mask can make the wearer appear intimidating. During Covid-19, patients of all ages had to adjust to seeing the faces of healthcare staff behind PPE. Would some of them become as frightened as plague victims who encountered Docteur de la Peste? It seems not, according to a study from Liverpool's Alder Hey Hospital, one of the UK's leading children's hospitals. Their work showed that PPE did not frighten children. On the whole, parents over-estimated the negative effects of masks. Youngsters between the ages of two and sixteen seemed reassured rather than traumatized, even when about to undergo surgery.

❧

What kind of mask is most effective? The N95 is one of the best, but there are many others. The Covid-19 pandemic saw the return of cloth masks, often homemade. While running them up out of scraps of fabric may have boosted *esprit de corps*, their efficacy is debatable. It's a difficult area to study, partly because there are few commercial cotton masks and no standardization of those made at home. Studies that include cottage-industry cloth masks are likely to find commercially manufactured disposable ones to be superior.

Single-use masks have obvious advantages. They're convenient, there are few labour costs, and sterility is guaranteed. A side-by-side comparison would seem almost unfair on the competition. Yet one piece of research found that a well-designed four-ply cotton mask can be just as efficient as a disposable one. It may even filter out micro-organisms more effectively after washing and drying.

If you've ever put something in the washing machine that you shouldn't have, you already know the fabric-tightening effect this can have.

I doubt disposable masks and respirators will ever disappear from clinical use. But, to reduce waste and pre-empt supply issues during a future pandemic – whenever that may come – it could be worth putting effort into developing effective reusable masks for the twenty-first century.

If someone's breath can carry disease, so can their hands. But protecting patients from infection was not the reason surgical gloves were invented. Two factors contributed to the evolution of gloves. One was a new treatment for rubber, pioneered in 1844. American chemist Charles Goodyear (1800–60) combined rubber and sulphur over a hot stove, a process that came to be called vulcanization after Vulcan, the Roman god of fire. The treatment stabilized rubber so that it could hold up to temperature extremes, which in turn enabled the production of a thinner, more malleable material that is nonetheless strong. Until then, gloves were made successively from animal caecum (part of the large bowel), cotton, silk, or leather, none of which was entirely satisfactory. In the early 1840s, pathologists sometimes wore strong rubber gloves for post-mortems but, being unvulcanized, these were thick and hard to manipulate.

The second major factor in glove evolution was the advent of antiseptic surgery (see Lister, Chapter 4). In 1867, Joseph Lister published his treatise *On the Antiseptic Principle in the Practice of Surgery.* Carbolic featured heavily in his recommendations. Other antiseptic agents included picric acid, iodine, and perchloride of mercury, all of which could trigger skin reactions. Despite this, surgeons still operated gloveless until the end of the nineteenth century.

Several doctors played a part in the development of modern surgical gloves, none looming larger than the celebrated American surgeon William Stewart Halsted (1852–1922). Having been a mediocre school student, he later found his calling and became one of the four founding fathers of the world-famous Johns Hopkins Hospital in Baltimore, Maryland, in 1889. As a surgeon, Halsted had excellent outcomes for the time. He practised an aseptic technique, and he handled tissues exceptionally gently, to traumatize them as little as possible. Among his many achievements was the operation of radical mastectomy that bears his name, although it has now made way for less mutilating treatments for breast cancer.

Halsted was bold as well as fastidious. When his sister nearly died from a massive haemorrhage after giving birth, Halsted swiftly drained off a large volume of his own blood and transfused it to her, then operated on her and saved her life. His treatment was one of the first emergency blood transfusions. In 1882, he carried out one of the first ever gall bladder operations in the US. It was 2 a.m., surgery took place on the kitchen table, and the patient was his mother. She too recovered.

Before long, Caroline Hampton (1861–1922) became the most important woman in Halsted's life. Hampton had been prone to dermatitis as a child. As the chief nurse in Halsted's operating theatre, she repeatedly had to plunge her hands in potassium permanganate solution, hot oxalic acid, and then in mercuric bichloride. These heavy-duty disinfectants made her skin condition return with a vengeance. Halsted considered Hampton an exceptional nurse. He felt he had to do something to protect her hands, so he commissioned the Goodyear Rubber Company to produce two pairs of thin rubber gloves made to measure from plaster casts of her hands.

The gloves were a success. Soon, Halsted's assistants began wearing gloves too, often declaring that they were more comfortable than bare hands. The outer surface of the gloves was textured, so it had the added bonus of making surgical instruments easier to grip. As for Hampton and Halsted, they married a few months later. Married women could not work, so Hampton did not wear her custom-made gloves for long. The Halsteds had dogs and horses rather than children, and were said to enjoy an eccentric lifestyle. Unfortunately, Halsted was addicted to cocaine, most likely from his work in pioneering it as a local anaesthetic. Later he became dependent on morphine as well.

Although assistants rather liked wearing gloves, surgeons continued to operate with bare hands for another seven years or so. Later, even Halsted was surprised that it took so long and commented that he must have been blind not to have perceived the need for gloves in the operating theatre.

One of Halsted's juniors noticed that gloves protected patients as well as staff. In 1899, the wonderfully named Joseph Colt Bloodgood (1867–1935) showed that using gloves during surgery reduced postoperative infection rates from 17 per cent to less than 2 per cent. Based on this, he insisted that the whole theatre team wear gloves. Bloodgood's nickname was Bloody, but in reality he was just as painstaking as his boss had been. His other important contribution to medicine was advocating health education of the public so that they could get an early diagnosis for conditions such as cancer.

The century or so since the first surgical gloves has seen a revolution in the rationale for them. Originally intended to shield staff from chemicals and later to protect patients from contamination by hands, nowadays gloves also safeguard staff from infections carried by patients.

Mikulicz-Radecki of Breslau began wearing a mask for operating in about 1897. Once he saw Halsted, he helped spread the glove habit. Others, too, ensured that gloves went worldwide. In England, Lord Moynihan was one of the first surgeons to use rubber gloves. At first, Berkeley George Andrew Moynihan (1865–1936) was mocked for it, as well as for changing into sterile white garments to operate. Some thought it was all a tad affected. He was also known for thorough handwashing and for introducing green towels in which to drape patients in theatre (green being less tiring on the eyes than white). As for himself, he denied ever being burdened in his life by tiredness. His colleagues agreed that he was not weighed down by modesty either. Moynihan was an exceptional surgeon, and he knew it.

Despite initial resistance to glove-wearing, it eventually became the norm. By 1920, gloves in the operating theatre were routine, although for some time nearly a third of trauma surgeons didn't wear them. As with all innovations, drawbacks emerged. First, surgical gloves needed to be sterilized. This made them harder to pull on, so powder was dusted inside the gloves to make it easier. A mixture of talc and other compounds was the most popular. A few years later, however, doctors began to diagnose granulomas in patients. These are areas of persistent inflammation, and they were often found inside the abdomen and other parts of the body that had been operated on. They could be painful, and they could mimic cancer.

By the 1940s, talc was recognized as the cause. It was replaced by corn starch mixed with magnesium oxide as a desiccant. But this new glove lubricant wasn't totally inert either. A few weeks after abdominal surgery, a patient could develop pain, fever, and vomiting due to starch granuloma peritonitis.

Powdered gloves were finally abandoned. Non-powdered latex gloves became the thing for operations and patient examination, and for animal surgery too. But rubber itself could cause ill health. Latex comes from the sap of the tree *Hevea brasiliensis* and contains hundreds of allergens with the potential to provoke serious allergy. The effects include skin reactions, asthma, and other breathing problems – even anaphylaxis, a severe reaction than can swiftly kill.

Of course, not everyone gets latex allergy. Those who've had five or more surgeries are most at risk, as are people with other allergies and those relying on daily procedures like catheterization. The at-risk group includes healthcare staff as well as patients.

Reactions to latex soared in the 1980s. It was a time when concerns about blood-borne diseases like AIDS led to the more widespread use of gloves for dental work and for simple procedures like taking blood. As a result, many more people came into contact with latex, and some became sensitized. Concerns over latex allergy then drove the switch to non-latex gloves, at least in the developed world. Alternatives to latex include deproteinized rubber, vinyl (PVC), polyisoprene, and nitrile. Nitrile gloves are often considered the best of those options, but they are expensive to the point of being unaffordable in many parts of the globe.

Needles, sharp instruments, or fragments of bone can pierce any glove, whatever the material. That's why surgeons may double-glove or even triple-glove when operating on patients who pose a higher risk of infection to others, especially for surgery that creates sharp surfaces such as tooth or bone. You may be wondering if wearing extra pairs of gloves is like operating with a catcher's mitt. As it happens, research suggests that it does not impair dexterity. Now that gloves come in a choice of colours, it's smart to wear the extra pair in a different colour, to show up tears more easily. And if a surgeon wants their hands to be as sensitive as possible, it pays to wear tight-fitting gloves rather than a size too large.

All PPE (personal protective equipment) comes at a price, and not just for the health provider. Medical waste is a growing challenge because so little is recycled. But, if they're not contaminated, latex, vinyl, and nitrile gloves can all be salvaged. Nitrile gloves could even play a role in the construction industry. When shredded, they bond well with cement, and adding a small percentage of shredded gloves can increase the strength of concrete by 22 per cent.

∞

No matter what covers the face and hands, it's hardly hygienic to operate in filthy smock encrusted with the blood and bacteria of previous patients. Yet that's exactly what surgeons of yesteryear did. Joseph Lister, no less, is said to have operated in his street clothes. When doctors wore anything to keep body fluids off their clothes, it was never sterilized, so it must have been disgusting and foul-smelling. No wonder most operations brought a heavy toll of infection and mortality until the late nineteenth century.

The advent of Pasteur and the germ theory (see Chapter 4, page 76) led to many improvements, one of them being the sterile surgical gown. The man usually lauded for its introduction is William MacEwen (1848–1924), who was a student of Joseph Lister in Glasgow and later followed him as professor of surgery there. His innovation was a gown made of fabric that could be laundered and sterilized. But MacEwen was not the only one of his day to develop a gown.

In Germany, surgeon Gustav Adolf Neuber (1850–1932) pioneered his own style of operating garb. He went further than Lister's thinking on antisepsis. In 1886, when he opened his own private hospital in Kiel, it was established on the principles of asepsis, in other words sterility. His clinic became known as the first aseptic hospital. Neuber decreed that surgeons and nurses had to wear long gowns stretching from the neck to the feet. Made of thin rubber, the gowns allowed the wearer to move, but they must have become unpleasantly warm. Fortunately, rubber gowns did not endure. Until sometime after the mid-twentieth century, most theatre gowns were made of cotton fabric. Then disposable gowns gradually took over.

Perhaps you can visualize the scene today, with a fully gowned and masked surgeon, standing in the operating theatre. He – because it's still more likely to be a man – also wears a cap over his hair. As he waits to begin cutting, he rocks on his heels in footwear kept exclusively for use in the operating suite – gumboots, clogs, or perhaps even Crocs. One shouldn't touch anything with gloved hands except the patient and sterile instruments, so, before the patient is wheeled in from the anaesthetic room, the surgeon may well clasp his hands together as if in prayer. At this point, there isn't much else to do. There may a brief comment to the waiting assistant or the scrub nurse, another roll of the eyes towards the clock on the wall, or perhaps a few impatient breaths, as seen in movements of the mask. Anaesthetists are rarely as speedy as surgeons would like, so the start of the operation may well be delayed. Then again, the surgeon might be praying not just for the anaesthetist to get a move on, but for a successful outcome, particularly if it's a challenging operation.

⚬⚬

White coats can function as protection for patients too, although that wasn't their initial purpose. In the nineteenth century, doctors began wearing white lab coats as a uniform to show that they were reputable scientists, in distinction to the many charlatans peddling their nostrums. Those working in labs wore them to protect themselves. Their white coats closed with buttons, and often had elasticated cuffs to avoid dangling a sleeve into a vat of something nasty.

When it came to working on hospital wards, a white coat helped keep the doctor's clothes clean. For the patient, the protective value depended on the coat pockets, which usually contained a stethoscope and vital reference works like *The House Officer's Guide to Medical Emergencies*. The hospital laundry often melted away every single button, but no matter. Flapping behind the young doctor as he or she strode to the next patient, the unbuttoned coat played its role in making a doctor appear more visible and more important.

Hierarchy is woven into the fabric, and the style of the white coat is often a crucial element of the semiotics. First-year residents at Johns Hopkins Hospital typically get short white coats that stop at the hip. Thereafter, they are allowed a coat that reaches to the knee. At some medical schools in the UK, both medical students and porters used to wear short white jackets. The only difference was that the students' version didn't have 'PORTER' embroidered in capitals above the breast pocket. Porters often arranged sheets of paper or a clutch of biros in that pocket to conceal their job description.

What do patients like physicians to wear? Research on 4,000 patients at ten academic medical centres in the US found that a doctor's attire influences how patients view their doctor, and even their level of satisfaction with the care they receive. On the other hand, white coats can be intimidating. In the UK, paediatricians, psychiatrists, and general practitioners gave up wearing them some time ago. Public preference depends to some extent on age. Younger patients prefer their physician not to wear a white coat, while patients over sixty-five prefer the opposite. Geography matters too. Patients in Denmark and the UK don't expect their doctor to wear white, while those in Sweden, Norway, and Finland do.

A doctor's garb can affect blood pressure, whether the patient is aware of anxiety or not. So-called white coat hypertension refers to situations where blood pressure readings are higher in the consulting room than elsewhere, such as in the patient's home. Although described as 'white coat hypertension' because many health carers wore white coats, it applies to any clinic setting. Some 15 per cent of the adult population exhibits the condition, and research suggests it may not be totally harmless.

The cleanliness of a practitioner's coat is obviously important. As Hippocrates urged in the fourth century BCE, physicians ought to be clean in person and well dressed. That isn't always the case. One memorable doctor of my acquaintance fell far short of this one weekend on call. He had been tinkering with his car when he was called to see a breathless patient, so he hastily donned a white coat and made his way to the ward. The nurse in charge had never met him before. She mistook him for the maintenance engineer and promptly showed him to a malfunctioning bedpan washer.

Whether or not they're worn in the sluice room, white coats carry germs. Research suggests that the cuffs and pockets are the most heavily contaminated parts, often with *Staph aureus* (in full, *Staphylococcus aureus*). The bacterial load depends on how much a coat is worn. How often should it be washed? Hospital laundries are no longer there to supply clean coats, so doctors increasingly have to wash their own clinical garb.

There may be little proof that white coats infect patients, but over the last few decades it has been impossible to ignore the soaring toll of hospital-acquired infections, especially those due to methicillin-resistant *Staph aureus* (MRSA) and *Clostridium difficile* (*C. diff*). Rapid patient turnover, low staffing levels, inadequate facilities, and the contracting-out of much hospital cleaning have no doubt played their part in the dramatic increase in MRSA. By the early 2000s, rates of MRSA in England and Wales had risen 600 per cent in a decade. With that in mind, the UK government decided to act. In 2008, it introduced a 'bare below the elbows' policy for doctors. Henceforth, there were to be only short sleeves, and no watches, rings, or neckties. Many hospital trusts soon encouraged the wearing of scrubs instead.

Since the early twentieth century, surgeons have worn scrubs, usually green, beneath their sterile gowns. These days, scrubs are also for physicians, nurses, medical students, health care assistants, and other clinical staff. This more democratic uniform may be clean and practical, but it also affects people's perceptions and can confuse patients and staff.

⚮

What of the future? The whole point of masks and other forms of PPE is to enable therapeutic interaction without risk to either party. Gloves and masks may continue to evolve and improve, but will they always be necessary? That depends on the future of medical practice. If virtual consultations and robotic surgery become the norm, we may not need protective barriers. Remote care is a world away from the traditional bedside manner, but it is already on the way. Whether it can meet the needs of both patient and doctor has yet to be seen.

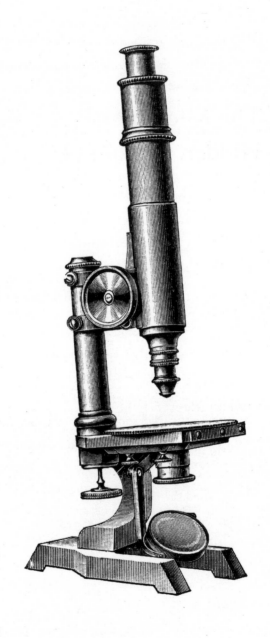

4

The Microscope and the Hidden World of Germs

Without the microscope, we would know nothing of microbes that cause so many diseases, and we would have next to no antibiotics. That's how important this object is. Vaguely lens-like objects go back millennia, but the earliest microscopes looked nothing like today's. They weren't even glass. Our forebears used crystals and water-filled spheres. Microscopes proper only came into their own when spectacle-wearing caught on in the thirteenth century. Those early, simple microscopes had just one lens and were barely more than a magnifying glass. So-called compound microscopes had two lenses, one near the object being viewed (called the objective lens) and another lens to view the image (called the eyepiece).

Physicist and astronomer Galileo Galilei (1564–1642) is most often – if not wholly accurately – credited as the inventor of the compound microscope. Sometime after 1610, Galileo realized he could tweak the focus of his telescope to examine small near objects. He began designing a compound microscope, apparently after being impressed by someone else's creation exhibited in Rome in 1624. That someone else was Dutch engineer and inventor Cornelis Drebell (1572–1633), so he deserves a mention.

The microscope remained something of a curiosity until the 1660s. Enter an Italian, a Dutchman, and an Englishman, who separately began using them for serious study. Italian biologist and physician Marcello Malpighi (1628–94) made detailed microscopic studies of various organs. He began with the lungs and small blood vessels of frogs. He also examined plants, insects, and humans. As a physician, Malpighi had an elite clientele and practised in several countries, often making diagnoses by post. You could think of him as an early adopter of remote consulting. He went on to care for his most illustrious patient when he became physician to Pope Innocent XII (1615–1700) in 1691. Today, Malpighi is immortalized in medical texts familiar to generations of medical students. Various anatomical entities, including renal corpuscles, nodules in the spleen, and a layer of the skin, are graced with the adjective Malpighian. It's no surprise that many consider him to be the Father of Histology (the study of the tissues of the body).

Born in Delft, Antonie Philips van Leeuwenhoek (1632–1723) was most definitely not the first microscopist. He wasn't even a scientist. A draper by trade, he established his own shop in 1654. He wanted to see in greater detail the quality of the thread, so he developed an interest in lens-making. He made small but superior lenses from strings of molten glass. He kept this innovation to himself, allowing others to believe that grinding, which he also used, was his only method.

Van Leeuwenhoek's most significant achievement lies in what he saw moving beneath his carefully crafted lenses. In 1676, he reported the discovery of microorganisms that he believed were tiny animals. Most of these 'animalcules' were, we now know, unicellular organisms such as bacteria and protozoa. He also studied multicellular organisms in pond water, as well as muscle fibres, sperm, and red blood cells. He was also the first to estimate bacterial size. His work led to the establishment of microbiology as a branch of science, and he is now commonly dubbed the Father of Microbiology.

Van Leeuwenhoek was a self-taught scientist who enjoyed working alone and distrusted others. Eventually, the Royal Society accepted his findings, but even so, many were sceptical of his discovery of microscopic life. Nobody had seen microbes before, and few were prepared to believe in them (although Jain scriptures from the sixth century BCE had hinted at unseen microbes). The belief at the time was that diseases came from the anger of the gods or from such things as poisonous air blowing across the Pontine Marshes (*malaria* literally means bad air).

A century earlier, Veronese physician and poet Hieronymus Fracastorius (*c.*1483–1553) had postulated that epidemics might spread via unseen seeds in the air, by direct contact, as well as through sexual contact, drinking water, and objects like clothing. There was plenty of support for his theory, since people discovered that they could develop conditions such as gonorrhoea from bedding the same woman as someone with symptoms. But nobody, Fracastorius included, appreciated that these seeds were also a form of life.

Van Leeuwenhoek changed all that. Although regarded as a hobbyist, he worked to an unusually high standard. It's likely that some of his microscopes could magnify up to 500 times. During his long life, he made over 500 optical lenses and at least twenty-five simple single-lens microscopes of different constructions. His single-lens microscopes were tiny, the largest barely as long as a thumb. They worked by keeping the lens close to the eye. The other side of the microscope had a pin to keep the sample near the lens. Screws moved the pin and the sample to change the focus, as well as to travel over differ- ent parts of the sample. Perhaps it was van Leeuwenhoek's commercial instincts that led him to keep his production method a secret. At any rate, for many years, scientists were unable to replicate his techniques.

Van Leeuwenhoek had studied muscle fibres at close range, so it was an unhappy coincidence that he developed uncontrollable muscular movements of his midriff, a rare condition now variously named van Leeuwenhoek's disease or belly dancer's dyskinesia. The involuntary contractions can be annoying and uncomfortable, but van Leeuwenhoek lived until the ripe age of ninety all the same.

Van Leeuwenhoek's contemporary, Robert Hooke (1635–1703), was not a medical doctor either. He deserves credit for being, along with van Leeuwenhoek, one of the first two people to discover microorganisms. He did so in 1665 with a compound microscope that he, too, constructed himself. That was only one of his accomplishments. Hooke worked as an assistant to the Anglo-Irish physicist Robert Boyle (1627–91), making vacuum pumps for his boss's experiments on gas laws. He branched out into constructing telescopes and microscopes, using them to study both planets and plants. His experiments led him to conclusions on the nature of light, the workings of gravity, the motion of the planets, and the effects of heat on solid matter.

A physicist, astronomer, and inventor, Hooke was also an architect, and he busied himself on the side with a little palaeontology, geology, map-making, watchmaking, and the study of memory. Some believe he invented the sash window, too. He was, one might say, a free thinker. At one point he fell out with the great Sir Isaac Newton (1643–1727) over universal gravitation. He also challenged the biblical version of the age of the Earth. It was Hooke who first described cells. He even coined the word 'cell' based on the resemblance he'd noticed between plant structure and honeycomb cells.

Microscopy had now revealed 'cells' and 'animalcules', but what did they actually do? Fast forward to the nineteenth century and Louis Pasteur (1822–95). Pasteur was a chemist and microbiologist, and arguably the most famous French biologist, as well as the most illustrious non-doctor in the history of medicine.

Early signs were inauspicious. As a youngster, Pasteur's main interests were fishing and sketching. He was an average student, until he discovered a passion for chemistry. Pasteur began studying fermentation in 1854, while dean of sciences at the University of Lille. Around that time, he made his famous comment that, in the field of observation, fortune favours only those with a prepared mind, or, as he put it, *dans les champs de l'observation, le hasard ne favorise que les esprits préparés.*

His studies led him to propose and develop modern germ theory. This was not immediately accepted (a recurring theme in relation to medical advances throughout history). A major hurdle was that Pasteur's conclusions ran counter to the doctrine of 'spontaneous generation', according to which living creatures could arise from non-living matter. This could supposedly be seen, for example, when maggots developed in dead flesh. No less a philosopher than Aristotle (384–322 BCE) had espoused spontaneous generation, and, as far-fetched as it may seem today, it had been regarded as scientific fact ever since.

With his experiments, Pasteur showed that foodstuffs spoiled because of contamination by invisible bacteria, not because of spontaneous generation. He developed a process of pasteurization, in which liquids were heated to a temperature of 60–100°C (174–212°F) to kill off most of the bacteria and moulds present. He patented the process in 1865 to combat diseases of wine. The method was later applied to lesser beverages such as beer and milk.

Fermentation received much of Pasteur's attention, too. He showed that yeast was necessary for alcoholic fermentation, and he elucidated how wine could go sour. His 1866 book *Études sur le vin* is a masterpiece on diseases of wine. Alongside this, he made significant advances in chemistry that later had an impact on human pharmacology.

Contamination of various drinks led Pasteur to conclude that bacteria could cause disease in animals and humans. He also encouraged doctors to prevent microorganisms from entering the body. We owe to him the foundations of hygiene, public health, and much of modern medicine. Despite being a chemist rather than a physician, Pasteur's work saved millions of lives through his discoveries in bacteriology and his development of rabies and anthrax vaccines. Quite simply, his germ theory changed the face of medicine.

Pasteur's body now lies in a vault in Paris beneath the Institut Pasteur, which he founded, and where he can be venerated daily. Many other cities all over the world also have streets that bear his name. Not surprisingly, there are also brewing companies named after him.

With Pasteur, hygiene was an idea whose time had come. Unfortunately, the medical world had not been ready just a few decades earlier. Ignaz Philipp Semmelweis (1818–65) was a Hungarian physician and scientist, and an early – too early, alas – proponent of antiseptic procedures in obstetrics. Puerperal fever or childbed fever was the name given to an infection many women developed after childbirth, and it was rife in nineteenth-century hospitals, killing many new mothers. While working as an assistant physician in Vienna General Hospital, Semmelweis observed that a certain delivery ward had several times the death rate of the other. On one ward, medical students arrived to deliver babies after coming straight from performing postmortems with dirty hands and instruments. The babies in the other ward were delivered by pupil midwives. In 1847, some ten years before Pasteur's germ theory, Semmelweis ordered that hands should be washed with chlorinated lime solutions. He didn't just dictate. He audited too. His publications showed that handwashing could reduce the death rate of puerperal fever to under 2 per cent. But his observations went against the established opinions of the day, and the medical community took against him and his ideas.

Colleagues were as offended as they were disbelieving. It would be a gross exaggeration to describe hospitals as hygienic in the mid-nineteenth century. Wards might be occasionally aired as a precaution against 'miasma', but medical men saw no need to wash their hands before attending to a patient, or at any other time. In those days, surgeons referred to the 'good old surgical stink'. The encrusted stains on their operating clothes were badges of honour and emblems of their expertise.

But Semmelweis could be trenchant in his views. In 1865, Semmelweis's colleagues committed him to an asylum. There he was beaten by guards and died two weeks later of a gangrenous hand wound, most likely from the beating. History has vindicated Semmelweis. Pasteur's germ theory was later able to provide an explanation for

Semmelweis's findings on puerperal fever. Years after his death, the doctor cast out by his colleagues was hailed as the 'Saviour of Mothers'.

∽⌁∾

Joseph Lister (1827–1912) was luckier. Many know of this surgeon as the Father of Antiseptic Surgery, but he made important contributions to physiology and pathology, too. Lister came from a wealthy family in Essex. As it happens, his father was a pioneer in the development of microscope lenses. There were no doctors in the family, but his father's scientific interests may have steered the young Lister towards medicine. As a Quaker, Lister was barred from attending the universities of Oxford or Cambridge, so instead he went to University College, London, where he gained a First.

Gangrene was rife when Lister was a junior surgeon. The procedure for dealing with a case was to chloroform the patient, scrape the slough off the gangrenous area, then burn the dead and dying flesh away with a mercury compound. The treatment sometimes worked. If, however, the edge of the wound produced a film and turned greyish, death was on the cards. Lister's boss believed that miasma was the cause of gangrene, but Lister was sure that it was something within the wound itself. He was vindicated when he looked at samples of gangrenous tissue through his microscope, finding things he had never seen before. Some kind of fungus, he suspected.

Lister studied Pasteur's papers while he was grappling with post-operative infections, and he became wholly persuaded that wounds became infected and purulent when microscopic airborne creatures settled in the wound. Lister decided to experiment on patients with compound fractures, meaning fractures where the skin is broken and bone ends might even poke out of the wound. If a treatment was found to work, it could be of great value with battle injuries or industrial accidents. He applied lint soaked in carbolic acid (also known as phenol). This did not always do the trick and, even when it did, it could irritate the skin. Carbolic was also smelly and flammable. Still, the results were encouraging enough for Lister to take the concept further.

He realized that a surgeon's hands, instruments, and dressings were all potentially contaminated with microbes. Therefore, while at Glasgow Royal Infirmary, Lister introduced the use of carbolic to sterilize surgical instruments, the patient's skin, the sutures, the surgeon's hands, and the operating theatre itself; in other words, pretty much everything in sight. Hygiene didn't, however, extend to the surgeon's outfit just yet.

Lister continued to develop improved methods of antisepsis and asepsis, and the death rate among his patients dropped from 46 to 15 per cent. Although he had become well known by then, not everyone agreed with him or his methods. Many surgeons simply took for granted that a large proportion of their patients would die.

Lister's best-known invention was the carbolic spray, first used in Glasgow in 1867 (and in many operating theatres throughout the 1870s and 1880s). Nicknamed 'the donkey engine', it was originally powered by a foot pump. The contraption weighed over 4 kg (8¾ lb) and delivered a pungent yellow mist of 5 per cent carbolic acid. It could provoke skin reactions, breathing problems, heart trouble, and even kidney damage for the surgeons exposed to it. Many became reluctant to use it, even though it made surgery safer for patients. Surgery using antiseptic established an important principle, and out of it grew aseptic techniques to stop microbes from reaching the wound in the first place. By 1887, Lister had given up carbolic spray for killing microorganisms in the air and concentrated on targeting them on instruments and dressings. He even admitted that he felt ashamed to have ever recommended his spray.

From today's perspective, Lister appears to have been a thoughtful and honest medic who built on the findings of those who went before him. He deserves his reputation as the Father of Modern Surgery.

It was Robert Koch (1843–1910) who took Pasteur's work forward and made further strides in the field of bacteriology. Koch was a German physician and microbiologist, and quite a stickler for rules. He also made some of his own. In 1882, he formulated criteria, revised and known today as Koch's postulates, that were necessary to fulfil to prove that a microorganism was the cause of a particular disease. One of the most important was that the organism must be present in every case of the disease. That sometimes took a lot of looking. But, assisted by the oil-immersion lens and the new techniques of culturing bacteria he had developed, Koch was a meticulous microscopist. With the aid of a microscope that his wife gave him, Koch showed in 1876 that anthrax bacilli (rod-shaped bacteria) were the cause of the disease seen in livestock. This was probably the first solid proof of germ theory.

More was to come. In 1882, he made his greatest single discovery when he isolated and cultured the tubercle bacillus. This was of monumental significance. Tuberculosis (TB) was, at that time, the largest single cause of adult death and killed nearly a quarter of the population of Europe. The work won Koch a Nobel prize in 1905. Later, when posted to Egypt, Koch also identified the bacterium that causes cholera.

TB continued to occupy Koch. Was there perhaps a substance that could stop the growth of tubercle bacilli and treat infected patients? He believed there was, and claimed that he had found it. He called it 'tuberculin'. Unfortunately, the stuff failed to live up to the assurances he'd given. It even killed some patients. When the tide turned against him, Koch fled to Egypt with a brand-new Mrs Koch. Rumour had it that he had already sold his TB remedy to a pharmaceutical company.

Although Koch was in disgrace, tuberculin did eventually serve a useful purpose, which he already suspected. When he injected it into himself, he developed a strong reaction. This, he said, proved he must have had 'a touch of tuberculosis' in the past. This is now the basis of the tuberculin test (in the form of the Mantoux or tine test). A vaccine against TB was eventually formulated in conjunction with the Institut Pasteur by Albert Calmette (1863–1933) and Jean-Marie Guérin (1872–1961). This is the well-known BCG or bacille Calmette-Guérin.

The rigorous new discipline of bacteriology led to major discoveries. In the late nineteenth century, microbes causing serious illnesses were identified at an average rate of one disease a year. They included diphtheria, typhoid, gonorrhoea, leprosy, plague, syphilis, tetanus, whooping cough, and streptococci (the bacteria that can cause scarlet fever and 'strep throat'). Many vaccines followed, for instance against typhoid. In the case of tetanus, the preventive measure was an anti-toxin serum, an antidote to the paralyzing toxin produced by tetanus bacilli. Vaccinations didn't necessarily depend on the isolation of the bacteria (or viruses) involved, but the knowledge certainly helped develop and refine vaccines.

<hr>

One of the most serious infections of all was, and still is, sepsis. It used to be called septicaemia as it is typically associated with bacteria in the bloodstream. However, that's not always the case, and the real cause of organ failure that leads to death in the condition is actually the body's overwhelming response to the initial trigger, which can be any of a range of bacteria or even viruses. The shorter name 'sepsis' may make the condition sound benign, but that couldn't be further from the truth. Without prompt treatment, the disease is deadly.

Once bacteria were identified, antibiotics could be developed that would work against sepsis and other life-threatening infections. German biochemist Paul Ehrlich (1854–1915) predicted pharmaceutical products that would target specific disease-causing organisms, hailing them as 'magic bullets'. He also carried out important work on the immune system, and was awarded a Nobel prize in 1908.

Penicillin heads the roll call of the first antibiotics, which includes sulphonamides, streptomycin, and isoniazid, which were very useful against TB as well as other microorganisms. Alexander Fleming (1881–1955) was a microbiologist at St Mary's Hospital, London. In the summer of 1928, Fleming was working on staphylococci, which are bacteria that can cause boils, impetigo, and more serious infections in those with compromised immunity. Before he left the lab for a two-week holiday, a petri dish with a culture of staphylococcus was accidentally left on a bench instead of being moved to an incubator as planned. It's not clear how mould got onto the dish. Popular retellings suggest Fleming left a sandwich on his desk. In reality, it's more likely that mould spores floated up in the air from the lab below. Anyway, the upshot was that, when Fleming returned in September, he found that a mould had inhibited the growth of bacteria in part of the dish. He also found that not all moulds did this, only some strains of *Penicillium*. Fleming named the active substance 'penicillin'. Thereafter, he carried out many more experiments. Howard Walter Florey (1898–1968) and Ernst Boris Chain (1906–79) followed up Fleming's discovery of penicillin, and the trio eventually shared a Nobel Prize in 1945.

Florey and Chain purified penicillin, then tested it on mice. Their findings in the *Lancet* in 1940 drew wide acclaim. With the world at war, the prospect of a cure for infections was especially appealing. In early 1941, Florey tested penicillin on humans. The first person had an alarming reaction due to impurities in the drug. The next was a forty-three-year-old policeman, Albert Alexander, who had developed sepsis from pruning roses. Alexander improved at first, but then relapsed. The supply of penicillin was scarce. Even salvaging penicillin from the patient's own urine failed to save him. Alexander died within five days. Henceforth, Florey promised, he would always ensure there was enough penicillin to complete a course of treatment. Of course, nobody knew the right dosage of the drug at the time or how long it should be used, but the outcome hints at the dangers of not finishing a course of antibiotics. The story also has another resonance. Some of today's drugs could save more lives, if only they were available in sufficient amounts to those needing them most.

Many more antibiotics have been discovered since, such as cephalosporins, first obtained from a mould near a Sardinian sewage outlet. Scientists search everywhere for potential new agents to treat bacterial infections. They've even looked into the secretions from the anal glands of the Argentine ant.

⤫

What of viruses? The study of viruses and the infections they cause began at the end of the nineteenth century. By then, Louis Pasteur and Edward Jenner (1749–1823) had already pioneered the first vaccines against viral illnesses, albeit without a clue that viruses existed.

Pasteur developed his vaccine for rabies from extracts of infected spinal cord, using rabbits then dogs as experimental animals. In 1885, he got his chance to treat a fifteen-year-old boy who had been bitten by a rabid dog. After fourteen days of painful daily injections, the lad survived, as did subsequent patients. This seemed miraculous, since rabies was almost always fatal, and still is today. Pasteur's vaccine spread widely. Celebrity followed.

Edward Jenner is the other big name associated with early vaccination success. Smallpox is a viral disease that has plagued humanity since Pharaonic times, if not before. It is said to have led to the downfall of the Aztec and Inca empires. A procedure called variolation was in use in England in the early eighteenth century. This involved transferring material from the pustule of a smallpox patient into a healthy person, usually with a lancet. Drawbacks included the risk of transmitting smallpox, even of triggering an epidemic, or just spreading some other disease from the blood of one person to another. Even so, inoculation seems to have been in use in several countries when they were faced with an imminent epidemic.

In 1757, eight-year-old Edward Jenner was one of many thousands of children to be variolated. It worked, giving him immunity to smallpox after just a mild dose of the disease. It also gave Jenner a lifelong interest in science. As a teenager, he was apprenticed to a surgeon and apothecary. One day, or so the story goes, he heard a pretty dairymaid say she would never get smallpox because she had previously had cowpox.

As in many legends, that's not what happened. The milkmaid version appeared in a biography of Jenner published a decade or more after his death, possibly to protect him against those who were adamant he did not discover the link with cowpox.

Jenner probably didn't. It's more likely that he heard of the link between cowpox and smallpox via a surgeon in the local pub. Jenner thought this over. Could cowpox be deliberately passed from one person to another in order to protect against smallpox? In 1796, he located a dairymaid called Sarah Nelms, who had fresh cowpox blisters on her hands and arms. Taking stuff he'd extracted from her blisters, he inoculated his gardener's eight-year-old son, James. The boy developed a mild fever, armpit discomfort, and appetite loss, but all this passed. Two months later, Jenner introduced matter from a fresh smallpox blister into James. He remained well.

We celebrate Jenner now, but he struggled to gain acceptance for this work at the time. Even when his vaccination became popular, he never made much from it, preferring to live modestly and vaccinate the poor free of charge in a hut in his Gloucestershire garden, a place many now consider to be the birthplace of public health.

Jenner achieved all this without any idea of what viruses were. Evidence for their existence first came from experiments with porcelain filters that had pores small enough to hold back bacteria but not viruses. Russian botanist Dmitri Ivanovsky (1864–1920) used such a filter in 1892 to show that sap from a diseased tobacco plant was still infectious to other plants even after filtration.

Dutch botanist and microbiologist Martinus Beijerinck (1851–1931) carried out similar experiments and later managed to replicate Ivanovsky's results. He was the one to name the filtered, infectious substance. His name for it was *contagium vivum fluidum*, which indicates the stuff is living and infectious. Beijerinck also acknow-ledged Ivanovsky's prior discovery.

Viruses are tiny (only 20–400 nm in diameter) and the vast majority can't be seen with a light microscope. That's because the resolution of an optical microscope is 500–1,000 nm, making only the largest, most complex viruses visible. Smallpox and cowpox viruses are among those, and can just about been seen with a light microscope.

Size isn't the only difference between viruses and bacteria. A virus is infectious, but it's only a segment of genetic material, either DNA or RNA, surrounded by a protein coat called a capsid. Sometimes the capsid has an additional spiky coat, called an envelope (as in the case of coronavirus, the appearance of which is famil-iar to most of us since the Covid-19 pandemic). Viruses latch onto host cells and get inside them, but they can't live or replicate on their own. They must use the host cell's equipment to reproduce. In so doing, the virus often kills the host cell. Each dying cell can release millions of new viruses into the body of the host, causing symptoms. It's worth knowing that viruses are able to linger outside the body for some time – for instance, on cutlery, door-knobs, or toys – which is one reason why doctors' waiting rooms can make you sicker. Many viruses cause diseases in humans, such as HIV, polio, Covid-19, measles, small-pox, and rabies. There are also more viruses that only infect plants or other animals.

Treatments against viruses have been more challenging to develop than those against bacteria, and no wonder. While drugs like penicillin and vancomycin, which break down cell walls in bacteria, can be powerful antibiotics, viruses are harder to reach as they live entirely within cells. So far, one of the most successful antiviral drugs has been acyclovir, which is active against several herpes viruses, including cold sores (herpes simplex) and shingles (varicella-zoster).

Viruses became more visible with the advent of electron microscopes. At the end of the nineteenth century, physicists became aware that the only way to improve on the power of the light microscope was to use radiation of a much shorter wavelength. Hence the electron microscope, which uses a beam of electrons instead of light.

In 1897, British physicist Joseph John ('J.J.') Thomson (1856–1940) discovered the electron, the first subatomic particle. Further groundbreaking advances in physics followed, many of them within the walls of Cambridge University's Cavendish Laboratory, where J.J. Thomson had identified the electron.

But back to medicine. In 1924, the aristocratic French physicist Louis de Broglie (1892–1987) showed that, when travelling in a vacuum, a beam of electrons behaves just like radiation of very short wavelength. In 1931, German physicist Ernst Ruska (1906–88) then managed to put these wave-like properties of electrons to use in the first electron microscope.

Two main types of electron microscopes are used for medical work, and both have a magnetic lens to focus high-voltage electrons onto a sample. The transmission electron microscope (TEM) uses a beam of electrons to pass through a sample. The scanning electron microscope (SEM) uses electrons finely focused to a point to scan across a sample. As a rough guide, TEM magnifies 50–50 million times, and the resulting image of the sample looks flat. SEM magnifies less, about 5–500,000 times, and the image looks sharp and three-dimensional. Sometimes TEM and SEM are combined in one instrument: the scanning transmission electron microscope (STEM). Electron microscopy has many uses, but one of the most important in medicine is to see inside viruses and other cells. Having said that, detecting bacteria and viruses these days relies increasingly on newer tests, like PCR (polymerase chain reaction).

Where are we now? The answer will keep changing but, thanks to the microscope, we now realize that microbes are everywhere, and they outnumber us. The average human contains about 38 trillion (38×10^{12}) bacteria and only 30 trillion (30×10^{12}) human cells. As for viruses, there are probably about 380 trillion (380×10^{12}) viruses in a body. Bacteria may be numerous, but they don't weigh much. In a 70 kg (11 st) adult, estimates for the total mass of bacteria range from 0.2–2 kg (½–4½ lb) which is only one of many reasons why taking antibiotics is not a good weight loss strategy.

Many bacteria are harmless. Some are even beneficial, like microbes that can keep the yeast *Candida albicans* at bay and prevent attacks of thrush. Scientists are also discovering how vital the bacteria and other microorganisms of the gut are to health. The gut microbiome is a unique community of trillions of bacteria, fungi, and viruses – unique because the community's residents vary enormously from person to person, even between identical twins. What this signifies is still emerging, but research so far suggests that the gut microbiome can heavily influence overall health, including immunity and mental health. Experts tell us to treat our gut microbiome kindly, but we probably need more insights and instructions as to how to do this.

Antimicrobials aren't always the magic bullets that Paul Ehrlich had in mind. They can knock out beneficial microorganisms, and they can also lead to antimicrobial resistance (AMR). Microorganisms resistant to common antibiotics are sometimes called superbugs, of which the best known is MRSA (methicillin-resistant *Staphylococcus aureus*). These can spread from person to person and lead to serious infections that can only be treated with difficulty, if at all. No wonder the World Health Organization calls AMR a threat to global health. Antimicrobial misuse is the main driver behind the growth of drug-resistant microorganisms. But it's a challenge to use them with pinpoint accuracy. Doctors often prescribe antibiotics before being sure which bacteria (if any) are responsible for their patient's condition. If rapid tests were available at the bed or desk, this might happen less. Wouldn't it be grand if there were a microscope and a microscopist wherever they were needed?

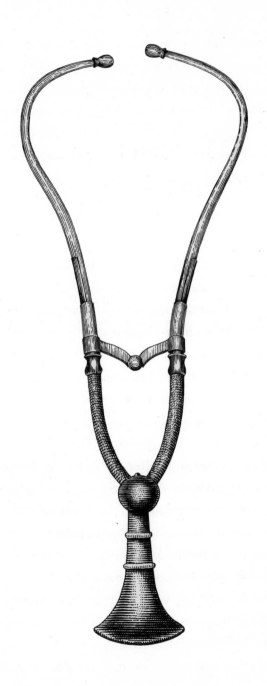

5

The Stethoscope: Listening to the Patient

~~∝~~

The most visible medical instrument of all is the stethoscope. Draped artfully across the neck, it announces that the person wearing it possesses special powers. As a rule, the wearer is the one most likely to believe in the near-divine significance of this badge of office.

In many ways, the stethoscope also ranks as the most important medical instrument. The object goes right back to 1816 and a young French doctor called René Théophile Hyacinthe Laennec (1781–1826). His surname comes from the Breton word *lennek*, which means scientist or expert, but is roughly pronounced *la neck,* which hints at where the device is most often kept.

Laennec was born in Quimper, Brittany. His father was a lawyer who was, unusually for the time, a vocal opponent of slavery. René's mother came from an aristocratic and highly musical family that included pianists and poets. Unfortunately, when René was just six years old, his mother died soon after giving birth to her fourth child, probably of tuberculosis. The baby died shortly after. The widower did not feel up to looking after his three surviving children, two boys and a girl. René was initially despatched to live with Uncle Michel-Jean, who was a priest near Quimper. But, when the uncle was called further away to a post in Tréguier, northern Brittany, René was parcelled off with his brother to another uncle in Nantes. By then, his father had remarried and there seems to have been no question of bringing the boy, aged about twelve at the time, back to Quimper. Uncle Guillaume (1748–1822) was a university rector and a doctor with a prestigious job at the hospital in Nantes. Just as important, he seems to have been a thoroughly decent guardian who was determined to educate René well and treat him like one of his own children.

⤜⤐

Many adolescents turn to musical instruments. So did René, though it was the flute he yearned to play rather than the guitar that modern teenage boys love. Recognizing the need for tuition, René wrote to his stepmother asking if he might be afforded an allowance for lessons. Thus far, financial help to the uncle had been on the erratic side, but, after some back and forth, his father substantially increased his contribution to his son's maintenance. René Laennec flourished. In addition to playing the flute, he threw himself into dance, art, poetry, choral music, and sport, including hunting. He was also an enthusiastic student of English, German, Latin, and Greek. Although he might have seemed destined for a career in the arts, his uncle's influence won out. The boy chose medicine.

Health was one stumbling block. Never a robust young man, Laennec also suffered at this point from a liver condition that today we'd probably call relapsing hepatitis. The other obstacle was the French Revolution. Simmering for years, revolt erupted in the late 1780s. The Bastille was stormed in July 1789 when Laennec was eight. This was followed in August by the Declaration of the Rights of Man and the Citizen. Inspired by Enlightenment philosophers, *la Déclaration des droits de l'homme et du citoyen* was a core human rights statement setting out the values of the revolution, which went on to make a major impact on events in Europe and the USA. It did not, however, ensure a peaceful transition of power from the king to the people, and bloody turbulence rolled on and on. In October 1789, a doctor called Joseph-Ignace Guillotin (1738–1814) proposed a new tool for public beheading, making for a swifter and more humane execution than hanging, drawing, and quartering. History tells us that the invention quickly made its mark.

Laennec's four years of medical education were punctuated by the revolution, during which he worked as a military medic in Nantes under his uncle's direction. He gained the rank of third-class surgeon at the Hôtel-Dieu in Nantes, which earned him a small stipend. Hôtel-Dieu is a common name for various hospitals around France that were founded in medieval times. The term originally meant 'hostel of God' in Old French; in other words, an establishment that received people in the name and under the auspices of God. Staffed by nuns, it took in beggars and pilgrims as well as sick people. The place was dilapidated in the extreme and teemed with patients and vermin. There was no guarantee of leaving alive, let alone healthy.

Guillaume Laennec was put in charge of completely renovating Nantes's Hôtel-Dieu. He increased the number of beds to 600 and housed them in wards with freshly whitewashed walls. The newly refurbished hospital was busy, especially given the fighting led by the Breton royalist, François de Charette (1763–96), in nearby Vendée. There were plenty of military casualties, and therefore many things for a novice doctor to learn. René Laennec soon became conversant with a range of clinical work, including wound dressings.

In 1801, he made his way to Paris to finish his studies. He was an excellent student. He also continued to play the flute and take part in chamber music recitals. By all accounts, he was a thin and sickly young man, no more than 1.6 m (5 ft 3 in) tall, but he had a powerful singing voice. Above all, he had the drive to succeed.

At that time, there were two main schools of medical thought. Jean-Nicolas Corvisart (1755–1821) was a well-known doctor and one-time physician to Napoleon who had a practical approach to medicine. Philippe Pinel (1745–1826), on the other hand, was a physician of a more theoretical bent. Laennec chose to follow Corvisart's teachings, studying anatomy in some depth. He doesn't seem to have warmed much to Corvisart as a person, not helped by the master's attempts to pass off Laennec's writings as his own. Still, Corvisart helped mould Laennec's thinking – and eventually got a Paris Metro station named after himself, too.

Laennec went on to become physician to the Salpêtrière Hospital in 1814, a vast establishment offering treatment to the poor. Thus he continued to gain a great deal of clinical experience.

⌒✕⌒

Like some of the best discoveries in science and medicine, the invention of the stethoscope was fortuitous. In late 1816, when Laennec was working in Paris at l'Hôpital Necker, he was called to visit a young woman with suspected heart disease. Laennec had already tried applying the palm of his hand, as well as percussing the chest, without getting any diagnostic clues. He was reluctant to put his ear on to the patient's chest because of her youth and *embonpoint*, which is to say large breasts. In this embarrassing moment, he picked up a notebook and rolled it up to form a tube that he then applied to the chest. To his delight, this enabled him to hear the heart more clearly than he ever had when placing his ear directly on to a patient's chest.

Why did it take over two millennia and any number of clever medics before anyone began listening to a patient's chest in this way? For one thing, nobody had any idea as to what caused disease. Around the time Laennec was born in the late eighteenth century, there were still outlandish theories about, such as the concept of the four humours inherited from Galen in the second century. According to this, every single body was composed of blood, phlegm, yellow bile, and black bile, and any form of ill health was due simply to an imbalance of these. Then there were those who believed in the contraction and relaxation of solid parts of the body, and yet others who maintained that living things couldn't be governed by the known laws of physics.

Although there had been some major advances, like William Harvey's (1578–1657) discovery of circulation in 1628, these had yet to revolutionize the practice of medicine. When it came to treatment, patients were either bled or purged. These methods were ineffective in epidemics and weren't much use for everyday diseases, either. When these therapies failed, patients were quick to seek supernatural remedies or to redouble their prayers to God. Life expectancy may have improved over the years, but it owed more to good agriculture and the absence of war than to medical know-how. Until the end of the eighteenth century, according to French physician and historian Paul-Marie Delaunay (1878–1958), medicine was little more than 'an ocean of ignorance in which bathed a few small islands of knowledge lost amidst myriad incorrect ideas'.

One of the striking things is that medical training of the time was very long even though medicine was near impotent against most diseases. Learning took place orally, with students taking notes on their knees. The professor was applauded like a showman when he entered and left the hallowed hall. Anatomy teaching was facilitated by a supply of corpses, although this became unreliable when executions stopped being a daily event. Teaching was tethered to the past and unlikely to be budged from it. Hippocrates was still considered close to God, and if something wasn't 'in Hippocrates' then it wasn't worth learning about. Clinical learning at the patient's bedside was non-existent. (By contrast, bedside learning is the hallmark of present-day medical schooling.) Patients of the past may not have benefited from all those years of study, but doctors looked older when they graduated, and it gave them a sense of importance far greater than their ability to cure anything.

Things began to change in 1794 with the creation of three *Écoles de santé* in Paris, Montpellier, and Strasbourg. Medical education became more practical with a new dictum: *peu lire, beaucoup voir et beaucoup faire* (to read little, to see a lot, and to do a lot). Still, at the end of the eighteenth century, doctors continued to assess their patients in more or less the same way as they had for centuries: they asked both patient and family extensive questions, then used their eyes. If they did occasionally feel for a pulse, it was not to count its rate but to opine on whether it was strong or weak.

For many years, it was considered rude for doctors to touch their patients. Instead, they would stare at the face and assess its general appearance and colour, then scrutinize the eyes and the tongue. Stools, phlegm, sweat, and blood were examined, and urine was inspected and smelled. Sometimes it was even tasted. None of this was considered ill-mannered. Why, it had been done since ancient times. (This was how, in 1673, Dr Thomas Willis (1621–75) had come to discover the sweet taste of urine in diabetics.) To some extent, these methods are still in use today, one difference being that doctors get lab technicians to deal with body fluids.

In the early nineteenth century, a sick person was an enigma. The only way to be sure of a diagnosis was to perform a post-mortem. As there were few effective treatments, this moment often came sooner than expected. French anatomist and pathologist Xavier Bichat (1771–1802) stressed the importance of a proper understanding of anatomy, pointing out that there was no substitute for looking and seeing inside a human body. He died after fainting at the Hôtel-Dieu hospital in Paris in his own basement labs. At the time there was no way of preserving corpses for dissection. A strong stomach and pipe-smoking were the only protection against the stench of putrefaction. Unfortunately, there was no safeguard against catching a dread disease from one of the cadavers.

Post-mortem suggested that Bichat had died of meningitis due to tuberculosis (TB), likely not helped by the treatment he'd received for fainting, notably leeches and an emetic. He was just thirty years old and had performed over 600 autopsies, making a detailed study of the tissues of the body. His ideas went on to influence Laennec, while his body went to rest in Paris's Père Lachaise Cemetery.

Despite this more anatomical approach, up until about Laennec's time it was rare to listen to the heart or the lungs (a method called auscultation). It had been mooted now and again, even by Hippocrates, but the idea had to bide its time.

Laennec's boss, Corvisart, was one early proponent of auscultation. He believed that diseases were being misdiagnosed on account of widespread ignorance of anatomy. Symptoms as described by the patient should correlate with anatomical findings at autopsy. Corvisart advocated placing an ear directly on the patient's chest, to better hear what might be going on inside. This technique was known as 'immediate auscultation', 'immediate' meaning the absence of any intervening media between ear and chest.

Other methods for examining the chest included succussion. This meant shaking the patient, much as you might shake a bottle of salad dressing to assess how much is left. If there was any fluid in the chest (or in your bottle of Heinz), it might produce a satisfying noise. In the case of chest fluid, however, the doctor had to shake the patient while keeping his ear on the chest. The method was sometimes useful, but it lacked finesse.

More sophisticated than succussion, a method called percussion was also in use, thanks to Leopold Auenbrugger (1722–1809). This Viennese doctor had, like Laennec, musical talents. He also happened to be the son of an innkeeper and had noticed his father tap a barrel with his fingers to tell if it was full or empty. Auenbrugger figured that the human chest was not so different from a wine barrel and, if tapped, would resonate if it was full of air (as it is meant to be when healthy). If full of fluid, the sound on tapping would be dull. Percussion is still done today, with the doctor placing their left hand onto the patient's chest and then tapping with the right middle finger onto the middle phalanx of the left middle finger.

It may have seemed an impromptu gesture when Laennec rolled up a notebook during his consultation with the young heart patient, but as he wrote in one of his papers, an event earlier that year had stayed on his mind. Walking in the courtyard of the Louvre, he'd watched two children sending signals to each other using a long piece of wood. With an ear at one end, one child received an amplified sound of a pin scratching the opposite end of the wood. Laennec might not have even noticed the children doing this had he not been of a musical bent.

Once Laennec realized how effective his simple roll of paper could be, refinements followed and led to versions in woods such as ebony, cedarwood, boxwood and lime. Laennec described the first stethoscope in a 900-page treatise published in 1819 entitled *Traité de l'auscultation médiate* – '*médiate*' because there was something interposed between doctor and patient. The two pieces of the instrument were screwed together and measured in total 4 cm (1½ in) in diameter and some 23 cm (9 in) in length. To get the best out of the apparatus, Laennec said it was to be held like a pen, and the doctor holding it was to keep his hand in close proximity to the patient's chest.

There was debate as to the right name for the new instrument. Suggested names included *sonomètre, pectoriloque, thoraciloque*, and so on. Laennec initially thought his invention to be too simple to merit a special name and just called it a baton. In the end, he settled on the name *stéthoscope*. *Stethos* meant chest in Greek, while *scope* referred to seeing inside it, although technically it enabled listening rather than seeing, unless one had a particularly vivid imagination. 'Stethoscope' did describe its main use, although Laennec predicted that it could also be used for parts of the body other than the chest.

Being just a wooden cylinder, the instrument had to be carried rather than worn. And it was. The French Revolution caused no shortage of injuries. Once it ended, other wars and revolts followed, right up to the Franco-Prussian War in 1871. Military medicine boosted the stethoscope's popularity. As armies travelled the world, they spread awareness of the new instrument to other countries.

Doctors from around Europe came to Paris to learn from Laennec how best to use this new instrument. British doctors were early adopters. In the 1820s you could buy a stethoscope in London for about four shillings (20 p). John Forbes (1787–1861), physician to Queen Victoria, translated *De l'auscultation médiate* into English.

It was published in London in 1821. Forbes said of the newly invented stethoscope, 'I have no doubt whatever … that it will be acknowledged to be one of the greatest discoveries in medicine.' A Prussian health officer took a stethoscope in his luggage to Japan, where it was swiftly reproduced in large numbers. Americans inevitably got in on the act and stethoscopes made in the USA soon hit the market.

It's not clear that Laennec received a *sou* from any of these sales. However, on home turf he had a number of eminent patients, among them the woman of letters Madame de Staël (1766–1817) and the author and diplomat Chateaubriand (1768–1848) and his wife, Céleste (1774–1847), who was also a celebrated writer. Unfortunately, de Staël died of heart failure, but the Chateaubriands enjoyed long lives, and continued to praise their little doctor.

With the aid of the stethoscope, the middle of the nineteenth century saw medicine gallop off in a brand-new direction. Now, instead of purging and bleeding, doctors applied science to their patients – even better, before they died. It was a momentous time in the evolution of medicine, and the stethoscope was at the beating heart of it. What was gleaned at the bedside could often be corroborated post-mortem. Speedy autopsies only increased the stethoscope's reputation.

Laennec was meticulous and modest. He built up a volume of detailed descriptions of what could be heard through the new instrument, classifying noises such as rales (now known as crackles) and rhonchi (now known as wheezes). He also described crepitation, a term still used today, even if modern doctors often scribble down 'creps'.

Aegophony was another of his findings. While rarely referred to these days, every medical student is taught that the term means sounding like a goat. The voice takes on a bleating quality when the doctor listens over an area of lung consolidation, as can occur in pneumonia. It can also be heard when there is fluid in the chest (pleural effusion) or lung cavitation. Typically, the patient is asked to say 'ee' while the doctor listens. In aegophony, 'ee' sounds more like an 'a'. Apparently, this is how a goat might say it.

Pectoriloquy literally means speaking with the chest. It refers to the transmission of a patient's whisper through the stethoscope via consolidated lung. The test may need to be done over different parts of the chest to discover which lung lobe is solidified. The patient therefore whispers 'ninety-nine' repeatedly as the doctor moves the stethoscope from one place to another.

Laennec applied the stethoscope to heart sounds, too, and described a variety of murmurs, some of which he considered rather musical. When he took a patient's pulse, he counted it like a true scientist with the help of a recently developed gadget, a watch with a hand for seconds. While Laennec's work on the heart was just as painstaking as his descriptions of lung sounds, his writings on cardiac findings did not endure. One problem was that patients found to have extensive calcium deposits in the heart valves at post-mortem did not always have abnormal heart sounds during life. Conversely, someone with a murmur heard at the bedside didn't necessarily have much to show for it at autopsy. Another reason was that Laennec, like other doctors at the time, believed the first heart sound to represent the beginning of diastole (the relaxation of heart muscle) and the second sound to indicate the start of systole (cardiac contraction). This is the exact opposite of what we know today.

∞

After studying symptoms and signs, and correlating the two, Laennec began a mammoth study of the diseases themselves, aiming to differentiate conditions such as whooping cough, bronchitis, and asthma based on what could be heard through his stethoscope. This was akin to using the instrument to visualize what was going on inside. It was also the first time serious scientific attention had been focused on individual illnesses.

He wrote an epic chapter on pulmonary TB. At the time, the disease was generally known as phthisis, which referred to its tendency to make patients waste away. Laennec studied the condition in depth and identified its hallmark finding as the tuberculous nodule. He believed all the manifestations of the condition to be variants of one single disease rather than many disparate disorders, as other doctors thought. However, he also believed heredity had a lot to do with its cause and did not consider the disease to be contagious. This was probably because so many members of his own family had died of TB.

Ever industrious, Laennec described various aspects of malignant melanoma in 1804, and was the first to give the name 'cirrhosis' to an affliction of the liver often linked with excess alcohol. One type of cirrhosis bears his name, but, perhaps strangely, the term 'Laennec's cirrhosis' is rarely used by doctors in his native France. In 1819, he was the first to describe the phenomenon of pulmonary embolism. It was not appreciated at the time how significant blood clots in the legs might be, but now it's well known that they can travel to the blood vessels in the lungs. That same year, having observed a sixty-seven-year-old man die suddenly, Laennec first used the term aortic dissection to describe a kind of tear that can occur in the aorta with fatal results. He also described the anaemia of lead poisoning.

Nowadays, we regard Laennec as a great pioneer of respiratory medicine and a moving force towards a more scientific approach to diagnosis. It wasn't always so. The birth of his more technical method was painful. You rarely get advances without complaints from those who prefer the status quo, and Laennec's invention duly had its detractors. Some thought it fanciful to believe so much information could come from listening with a tube. Many pointed out that none of the findings had any bearing on whether the patient would improve. And a few simply found fault with the name 'stethoscope'.

They could not have imagined that a stethoscope can now help doctors diagnose pneumonia, pleural effusion (fluid in the chest), asthma, lung fibrosis, pleurisy, heart valve disease, heart failure, and pericarditis, to name just a few conditions. A stethoscope is also useful for picking up arterial bruits. These are a kind of murmur caused by turbulent flow in a large blood vessel, for instance, when a carotid or femoral artery is partially blocked. And, with a stethoscope applied to the belly, a medic can also detect the tinkling bowel sounds of gut obstruction or the silent abdomen of peritonitis.

Stethoscopes are also used to measure blood pressure. An Italian physician and paediatrician, Scipione Riva Rocci (1863–1937), is credited with the invention of an easy-to-use version of a device to measure blood pressure in the 1890s. Now commonly abbreviated to 'sphyg', the sphygmomanometer has a glass column of mercury connected to Riva Rocci's innovation, a flexible cuff that goes around the arm of the patient. Crucially, this method requires a stethoscope positioned over the brachial artery at the front of the elbow crease. The cuff is inflated until the medic can no longer hear the pulse over the artery. Then, deflating the cuff slowly, the moment the pulse is heard again marks the patient's systolic blood pressure. Letting the cuff deflate further eventually leads to a point where the sound can no longer be heard. This is the diastolic pressure. The mercury sphyg has now fallen out of favour because of its mercury content and has been all but replaced by digital instruments that don't need a stethoscope. Even so, blood pressure is still recorded in millimetres of mercury, with the systolic figure as the numerator and the diastolic as the denominator, as in 140/80.

∽

A few years after its first appearance, the stethoscope began to morph. British physician Golding Bird (1814–54) described using a flexible tube as a stethoscope in 1840, though it's likely that there were previous similar models. In 1851, Irish physician Arthur Leared (1822–79) claimed to have invented a stethoscope with two earpieces. Then again, that accolade might go to fellow Irishman Nicholas Comins (dates unknown), who, it's said, described a binaural design as early as 1829. It had brass tubes connected by moveable joints with coiled silk inside the joints to make them airtight. In 1852, New Yorker George Phillip Cammann (1804–79) perfected the binaural instrument, and that became the template for commercial models ever since. Subsequent designs incorporated increasingly long tubes to make life more convenient for both doctor and patient without compromising sound quality. On the whole, however, the longer the tube, the less faithfully sounds are transmitted.

As used today, a regular binaural stethoscope generally has two heads, one a bell made of stainless steel and the other a diaphragm with a resin membrane. The diaphragm picks up higher pitched sounds. Both heads have non-metal rims so that the instrument doesn't feel cold on the skin. Since the tubing is narrow, sound vibrations are funnelled upwards instead of dissipating as they would without an instrument. Each sound wave bounces off the inside walls of the tubing, which amplifies their effect. Lower pitched sounds are slightly different in that they cause vibration of the skin, and these are best detected with the bell. In fact, the diaphragm can miss some low-frequency sounds.

In the early 1960s, US cardiologist David Littmann (1906–81) patented a design that hugely improved the acoustics of the stethoscope. In 1967, 3M acquired his company and took on Littmann as a consultant. These days, the 3M Littmann is the gold standard in stethoscopes, with some models, like the Cardiology IV, costing £200 or more. It has a tuneable diaphragm so that the doctor can hear sounds of different frequency.

You can also have your initials engraved on the stethoscope to reduce the risk of your investment going walkabout. A more common, if less elegant, way for doctors to stake their claim on their stethoscope is to wrap a plastic patient ID wristband around it, with their name scrawled on it in biro. Currently, most stethoscopes are black, grey, or dark blue, but they come in many other colours. An eye-catching red or purple can make the instrument less likely to go astray.

There's also a choice of stethoscope model for every medic. The usual design has a single tube leading to the chest-piece, but the Sprague-Rappaport stethoscope, designed in the 1940s, has two shortish tubes that lead from the stethoscope chest-piece to the curved metal earpiece. Held together with metal clips, the dual-tube arrangement is heavy and has an old-school look but gives superlative sound quality. While not everyone finds it comfortable to use, it remains a good choice for would-be cardiologists, and the head can be changed to a more compact one for use on children.

Paediatric doctors need instruments that are in proportion with their patients. A paediatric stethoscope has a smaller head for auscultating small patients. A snazzy colour can make it more child-friendly. It also helps if the doctor listens to a teddy bear's chest first.

You could be tempted to consider the fetal stethoscope to be an extreme variant of the paediatric instrument, but, with its simple conical shape, it is very different. Also called a Pinard horn or just a Pinard, it was invented by French obstetrician Adolphe Pinard (1844–1934) in 1895. He was a leading light in antenatal and maternal health, and he developed methods for examining women in labour. There is no Metro stop named after him, but he does have a Paris boulevard to his name. Even better, midwives all over the world use his invention.

Electronic stethoscopes work by transforming sound vibrations into an electronic signal and can amplify sounds up to twenty-four times. Some of the models have noise-cancelling properties. Some can also store short tracks or have apps to display the audio data visually. Electronic stethoscopes can transmit data via Bluetooth. Some hearing-impaired medics manage with an electronic stethoscope, but others need other digital solutions, especially if they wear hearing aids. Yes, there are stethoscopes for them too.

❧

Microorganisms were unknown in Laennec's day, but they caused much ill health at the time, and infections still loom large in modern medical practice. Anything that might increase the risk of healthcare-acquired infection has come under scrutiny, which is one reason why ties have become passé for doctors. The other is the rising number of women doctors. Like the doctor, a stethoscope also travels from patient to patient, and research shows that the instrument often carries bacteria such as staphylococci, pseudomonas, MRSA, *E. coli*, and *Clostridium difficile*, as well as a number of less harmful microbes. Studies have found that a stethoscope carries about as many bacteria as a doctor's dominant hand – one more reason to consider the instrument as the medic's 'third hand'.

Many consultations are short, though not quite short enough to prevent transmission of microbes from a stethoscope to a patient's skin. Experiments show that it takes just three seconds of contact, whereas listening to the chest typically involves several minutes of skin contact, and thus ample time for germs to transfer. If germs can travel one way, they can make the return trip, too.

A solution of 70 per cent ethanol wiped onto the instrument between patients might be a good decontaminant, but, in real life, very few doctors or nurses clean their stethoscopes regularly, if at all. Some authorities have suggested the use of disposable aseptic barriers. Others have proposed disposable stethoscopes, but these are poor substitutes and have even led to misdiagnoses.

What's to be done? Reassuringly, so far, the stethoscope only seems to have the potential to spread infection. It's not been proven that it actually does so. Skin is usually an effective barrier, as long as it's intact.

❧

Technological advances mean that patients nowadays are not always examined fully before they get an X-ray or some other tests. What is the point, ask some, of percussing the chest, then listening carefully with a stethoscope and possibly checking for exotic signs, such as whispering pectoriloquy, if the patient will be sent for an X-ray, regardless? Good question, but tests take time, cost money, and can have drawbacks. Unthinkingly applying technology doesn't always serve patients well and it can be a drain on resources.

No matter how fancy the stethoscope, the most important part remains the bit between the doctor's ears. As a rule of thumb, breath sounds are easier to make sense of than heart sounds. Expertise in listening to the heart takes longer to acquire. For the past fifty years or more, there have been new and painless diagnostic methods for heart disease, such as echocardiography, hand-held ultrasound, and MRI. Using a stethoscope to auscultate the heart has begun to fall by the wayside, and few doctors are now taught in depth how to use it.

Even so, it's safe to say that, more than 200 years after its invention, the stethoscope remains valuable, cost-effective, convenient, and patient-friendly. Its deployment reassures a sick person that they are being taken seriously and literally being listened to.

⁓

Back to Laennec himself. By all accounts, he was intelligent, patient, hardworking, devout, and lucky – except when it came to his health. He was often breathless from asthma and grew thinner over the years. In 1824, he married a widow, Jacquette Guichard Argou. To their sadness, her one pregnancy came to grief. During his last few months, he asked his nephew Mériadec Laennec (1797–1873), also a respected physician, to listen to his chest. Mériadec's description was alarmingly familiar. Finally, Laennec believed what he had denied for so long; he too had cavitating TB, and it would soon claim his life. When Laennec died in 1826 at the age of forty-five, he left all his scientific papers to Mériadec, as well as his ring, his watch, and 'above all, my stethoscope, which is the best part of my legacy'.

The stethoscope remains the very emblem of a doctor. Laennec's legacy, however, is even greater than his stethoscope. For the first time, instead of relying on woolly and unverifiable theories of disease, doctors began to apply a truly scientific method to assess their patients.

Laennec was something of a pioneer in other ways, too. He was never arrogant or keen to dazzle with his brilliance. Nor did he just listen to patients with the aid of his tube. He sat beside them as they shared their concerns with him. He knew that social and economic factors could be important in disease, too. René Laennec was, in short, patient-centred in every sense of the term.

When medical students first acquire a stethoscope, they invariably hold themselves a touch straighter, stand a little taller, and stride down the hospital corridor with greater confidence. But a stethoscope draped around the neck should also remind its wearer to aspire to the best qualities of a doctor.

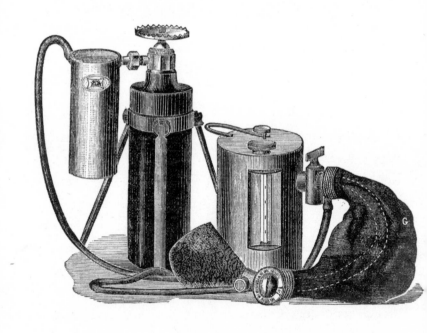

6

The Ether Inhaler and
the Conquest of Pain

Pain has been with us since humanity's earliest days, if not much earlier, since our animal ancestors must have suffered it too. Efforts to relieve pain, whether due to disease, trauma, or surgical intervention, also go back a long way. Opium, alcohol, and mandrake were used in antiquity. In the Middle Ages, the anaesthetic might have been a sponge soaked in opium, henbane, mandrake, lettuce, or mulberry. By the mid-seventeenth century, gin, whisky, and rum were favoured painkillers. The techniques were often harmless, though not always. One tactic was to induce a head injury to bring on a blessed loss of consciousness.

More acceptable strategies took a while to arrive, and even longer to be recognized as valuable. Ether (or to be exact, diethyl ether with the formula $C_4H_{10}O$) was first synthesized in the thirteenth century. But it was only much later that it was used for pain relief or sleep.

There was a passing fashion for mesmerism in the early nineteenth century. This method and the closely related concept of animal magnetism came from German physician Franz Mesmer (1734–1815). When it worked as a method of pain relief, which was far from assured, it probably did so by hypnosis or by the power of placebo. For some time, though, it was one of the few methods available.

The first effective anaesthetic drugs to come into use all worked by inhalation and had nothing to do with hypnosis or with those early herbal preparations. They were nitrous oxide (N_2O), ether, and chloroform ($CHCl_3$), and they came about as a result of the Enlightenment, when British scientists identified several gases. Between 1754 and 1772, chemist Joseph Black (1728–99) discovered carbon dioxide, while chemist and theologian Joseph Priestley (1733–1804) discovered oxygen and nitrous oxide. In 1799, chemist Humphry Davy (1778–1829) – the inventor of the Davy lamp – spotted that nitrous oxide caused euphoria when inhaled. He came up with the term laughing gas and also suggested that it might work as an anaesthetic for surgery. Nobody took much notice, however, so he kept himself busy with other things like isolating chemical elements and writing poetry. A little later, scientist Michael Faraday (1791–1867) joined Davy, and they looked into ether rather than nitrous oxide, publishing some of their observations. Unfortunately, one of their observations was that people could take twenty-four hours to recover from its effects.

For a while, the use of both ether and nitrous oxide remained purely recreational. 'Ether frolics' and laughing gas parties were popular. People would sniff it, become giggly and giddy, then collapse, all of which was deemed socially acceptable. The term laughing gas persists today, and teenagers still use it for fun, unaware that it can cause serious trouble. Crime statistics for the early 2020s showed that nitrous oxide was the second most commonly taken recreational drug among sixteen to twenty-four-year-olds in England, the first being cannabis. Those working in emergency care report that abuse of nitrous oxide plays a large part in Accident and Emergency visits in this age group. Discarded cylinders left on street corners can be cleared up. The damage that excess nitrous oxide can cause to the spinal cord is more permanent. Nitrous oxide is now a Class C drug under the Misuse of Drugs Act 1971, making possession and sale for recreational use a criminal offence.

~×~

Despite its contributions to many other areas of medicine, France does not feature much in the history of anaesthesia. The exception is the notable French chemist Antoine Lavoisier (1743–94), who is credited with understanding the importance of oxygen in the seventeenth century. He also made possible many other advances in chemistry and physics that are indispensable to modern medicine. Of course, oxygen is not a painkiller, but it is essential to life, whether you're climbing a mountain or lying on an operating table.

Most of the story unfolds in the US, with several Americans making contributions that eclipsed those from the rest of the world, at least to begin with. I say unfolds, but it is a convoluted tale full of rivalries and disputes.

At times, it's difficult to be sure exactly who was responsible for which discovery. It's usually accepted that, in 1846, dentist William Morton first demonstrated that inhaled ether worked as an anaesthetic. But there's more to this account than meets the eye.

Morton's part in the story starts in Hartford, Connecticut. In 1844, a travelling showman by the name of Gardner Quincy Colton (1814–98) gave a demonstration of nitrous oxide. In the audience was dentist Horace Wells (1815–48). His particular skill was fashioning dentures. Having seen Colton perform, Wells immediately thought nitrous oxide could benefit his dental practice because, before supplying dentures, the patient's rotten teeth needed to be removed. Wells decided to begin with the extraction of one of his own upper molars. The very next day, he put his trust in the showman and his nitrous oxide, and opened wide.

Impressed with the outcome, Wells learned to make nitrous oxide, and then passed on his experience to his Harvard student, William Morton (1819–68), who later became his colleague in dental practice. It was Morton who saw the need for something better and longer lasting than nitrous oxide.

What about Wells? His brain may have been damaged from self-experimenting with ether and chloroform. At any rate, he left dentistry and began selling shower baths. In 1848, he was arrested for throwing sulphuric acid over the clothes of two ladies of the night in New York. Soon after that, he deliberately slashed his femoral artery with a razor and died in jail. He was thirty-three.

Colton the showman thrived. He continued for a while with his demonstrations and with giving nitrous oxide for dental extractions. Eventually he gave up his shows and set up a company specializing in tooth-extraction services. Meanwhile, Morton, the biggest player in this tale, more or less abandoned nitrous oxide and began experimenting with ether. He consulted his chemistry teacher, Charles Jackson (1805–80). This appears to have influenced Morton but it's uncertain to what extent.

When Morton was satisfied with his work on ether, he was ready for a real-life demonstration. The operation on 16 October 1846 was the removal of a tumour from the neck of one Gilbert Abbott. In front of a large crowd, John Collins Warren (1778–1856), surgeon at the Massachusetts General Hospital, operated while Morton administered ether vapour to Abbott. The patient showed not one sign of distress.

The era of painless surgery had dawned. The ambitious Morton realized it, and there was no stopping him. With an eye on his own future, he hoped to lay claim to the discovery of anaesthesia. He aimed to profit from ether by patenting it, all the while calling the stuff 'Letheon' and adding colourant to dupe his colleagues over the identity of the vapour he'd used. But they were not that gullible. Morton and his old chemistry mentor Charles Jackson fell out and became sworn enemies.

The animosity probably wasn't all one-sided. Jackson also managed to quarrel with others over the discoveries of guncotton and the telegraph. Finally, peace reigns, with both Morton and Jackson interred in the same cemetery in Cambridge, Massachusetts.

The only thing wrong with this version of events is that, in reality, a pharmacist and surgeon from Georgia, USA, got there about four years before Morton. Crawford Long (1815–78) used ether for the first time in March 1842 when removing a tumour. He poured ether onto a towel and got the patient to inhale it. He performed several similar operations but, unfortunately for him, he didn't publish anything until 1849, so Morton got the credit.

There is a monument to ether in the north-west corner of Boston's Public Garden. Also called the Good Samaritan monument, it dodges the whole issue of priority of discovery by depicting a Moorish doctor holding a patient. The granite bears biblical and other inscriptions but has no name on it – not Wells, Morton, Jackson, or Long.

Once that landmark surgery under ether took place in Boston in 1846, things moved rapidly. News of Morton's success with ether crossed the Atlantic. In December that year, surgeon Robert Liston (1794–1847) used it to great effect for an amputation. This wasn't the first use of ether in Britain, but it is the most celebrated. Interest in pain-free surgery grew apace. The next trio of notable doctors of the time were British and had the given names James, John, and Joseph, respectively.

First up, James, by which I mean James Young Simpson (1811–70), an obstetrician from Edinburgh. He had taken lectures delivered by Liston, and had been duly impressed. But Simpson realized that ether had draw-backs. For one thing, it made patients nauseated. For another, the vapour was flammable, making it risky in the days of gaslight.

Simpson and his friends decided to try other agents. While seated at dinner, or so the story goes, they sniffed various drugs. When they tried chloroform, the mood was light and frivolous. But soon they all collapsed, as Mrs Simpson discovered when she came in. Some of the party remained inert until the next morning.

Whether Simpson really tried chloroform around the table with his friends is up for debate. He probably wasn't the first to discover the drug. However, he did appreciate its value, and he became enthusiastic about pain relief in labour, which is one of his greatest contributions to medi-cine (see also Chapter 8, page 173).

Next comes John Snow (1813–58), the first doctor who could be called a specialist anaesthetist. It's doubt-ful whether this son of a labourer from York could have afforded to study medicine at all had it not been for a wealthy uncle. Even then, Snow had to walk 645 km (400 miles) to reach London.

Once in practice, Snow quickly understood that mishaps could arise if the most junior people were left to give anaesthetics, which is what happened at the time. What's more, it was impossible to assess the dose of ether inhaled. In 1847, Snow designed an apparatus to dispense ether safely. His ingenious device used a hot water bath under the ether bottle. The temperature of the water regulated roughly how much ether vapour was produced, and so how much the patient inhaled via the wooden face mask that was part of his apparatus. The mask also had a mouthpiece for the patient to bite down on. Soon the entire practice of ether, in London anyway, was in his hands, and it was a lot safer for it. When chloroform came into use, it proved faster than ether. It was also non-flammable. Snow quickly adopted the drug and also designed a mask to administer it. He appreciated that chloroform, being more potent than ether, should be even more carefully used.

One tragic example is that of a fifteen-year-old girl named Hannah Greener. All she had wrong with her was trouble with a toenail. In January 1848, she had the nail removed in her home under chloroform. The drug was not measured in any way. It was simply poured onto a table-cloth and held onto the girl's face. But her heart stopped and she never recovered. This was the first recorded fatal-ity due to anaesthesia. Snow investigated this case and the deaths that followed, which became one of the first peer reviews in the new speciality. Hannah had died, he concluded, because the dosage of chloroform was uncontrolled. In future, scientifically engineered vapor-izers had to be used.

The pinnacle of Snow's career was being summoned to dispense chloroform to Queen Victoria in 1853 for the birth of Prince Leopold, and again in 1857 for the birth of Princess Beatrice. He is said to have used a silk handker-chief to administer the vapour. At the time, many eminent doctors were against pain relief in labour – as was the Church – especially for a normal labour. However, the queen endorsed it, and who could argue with that? Soon, everyone was talking about *chloroforme à la reine*.

Snow's other claim to fame is his work in epidemiology, specifically in tracing cholera outbreaks to contaminated water. Nobody believed him at first. Doctors and everyone else were convinced that disease came from miasma (the stench from rotting animals and vegetables). Snow persuaded himself, if not others, of the origin of one outbreak in London's Soho by removing the handle of the water pump in Broad Street that he'd identified as the source of the outbreak. This led to a decline in cholera cases. Snow was a vegan and teetotaller who campaigned for temperance societies. One can only imagine what he might have made of a pub named after him. The John Snow is in Broadwick Street – the current name for Broad Street – and right beside it stands a replica water pump.

Snow died at the age of forty-five, a year after he last gave chloroform to the queen. He was not a well man, and possibly never was. In his youth he had had TB of the lung. Later he may have developed kidney failure linked with exposure to anaesthetics. He had investigated almost every possible compound that might be a useful anaesthetic, often experimenting on himself, as did most scientists of the day. At the time, of course, the side effects of most of the drugs weren't recognized. Today we know that chloroform can harm the skin, the eyes, the liver, the kidneys, and the nervous system. It can also cause cancer.

And finally for the Joseph of this story. Joseph Clover (1825–82) was a shopkeeper's son from Norfolk who went to study medicine at University College Hospital, London. After graduating, he initially went into surgery, then left it for general practice which better suited his fragile health. From there, he developed an interest in anaesthetics where he made his mark. The death of John Snow in 1858 had left a void, and Clover filled it by becoming a 'chloroformist' for several London hospitals. He and his patients were lucky. By 1871, Clover had given chloroform some 7,000 times and other anaesthetics about 4,000 times, apparently all without a fatality. In 1874, however, a patient of his did die after chloroform anaesthesia.

Anaesthetic drugs were a great improvement on being clubbed senseless over the head, but they have always been a two-edged sword. Too small a dose, and the patient will be awake in pain. Too large, and the patient may not leave the operating theatre alive. At that time, the success of a treatment was attributed entirely to the doctor involved. But Clover understood that skill alone is not enough. The outcome also relies on the right equipment. In 1862, he designed a chloroform apparatus, and in 1877 he made one for ether. His ether inhaler was the first apparatus that properly regulated the amount of ether inhaled. It incorporated a small dome-shaped reservoir and a dial to regulate the percentage of air that passed over the ether. It was portable too, enabling the doctor to take it to whichever hospital called for their services. Since then, his ether inhaler has been updated, and it lasted, with modifications, until well into the twentieth century.

Like Snow, Clover treated VIPs. He administered anaesthetics to no less than Napoleon III of France (Napoleon Bonaparte's nephew), Edward VII (as Prince of Wales), his wife Alexandra of Denmark, Sir Robert Peel, and Florence Nightingale. Whether you consider that these illustrious people match the celebrity of Queen Victoria is a personal judgement.

Clover understood that the effect of nitrous oxide was too short-lived except for the quickest procedures. However, he thought it could be useful for speeding up the action of ether, for instance to induce anaesthesia. He effectively began the trend for deploying a combination of different drugs, which reduces the risk of side effects from using large doses of just one single drug. This multi-drug approach is current practice, and can be considered another of Clover's great contributions. Alongside Snow, he is immortalized on the crest of the Royal College of Anaesthetists, and he is buried in Brompton Cemetery, London, also not far from Snow.

❧

Anaesthetics were not just for the rich and famous. They were for soldiers too. The American-Mexican War of 1846–8 saw the first anaesthetics given for surgery, such as amputation. While patients may have approved, not everyone believed pain-free surgery to be a good thing. Many mid-nineteenth century surgeons were convinced that more patients died if the operation took place under anaesthesia.

US Army surgeon John B. Porter (*c.*1810–69) was one of them. He adamantly opposed the use of anaesthesia. He professed to worry about a tendency to bleed and adverse effects on wound healing. Neither of these fears was real, but it did not stop him imposing his beliefs on his men and prohibiting the use of anaesthesia under his command. Porter's views also reflected the rigid concepts of masculine bravery that existed at the time. If pain didn't build a young man's moral fibre, what did?

By the way, the phrase 'to bite the bullet' may come from a soldier clenching a bullet between his teeth to deal with the pain of surgery, but in reality it was more usual – and a lot less damaging to teeth – to bite on a leather strap during an operation.

In time, things did change. When the American Civil War broke out in 1861, ether and chloroform had both been in use for several years. At this point, chloroform came out as the front-runner because it worked more quickly. Inevitably, military medics on both sides of the conflict had to carry out many, many thousands of operations, most of them amputations. Chloroform became an indispensable drug. In much the same way, the British Army almost exclusively used chloroform during the Crimean War (1853–6).

The First World War and the scale of the trauma inflicted drove further advances. Irish-born Ivan Whiteside Magill (1888–1986) was an anaesthetist who worked alongside the pioneering reconstructive surgeon Harold Gillies (1882–1960) at the Queen's Hospital, Sidcup, Kent. The horror of the injuries of the Great War was matched only by Gillies's resourcefulness in dealing with them. Magill had to be equally creative because it was impossible to use a conventional mask for giving chloroform or ether to servicemen who'd suffered severe facial injuries. In 1919, Magill and his team developed tubes for inserting directly down into the trachea to deliver anaesthetics. Magill gave his name to several medical devices, most of them vital to modern anaesthetic practice.

⚬⚬

The need for a more rapid onset of anaesthesia led to a search for injectable drugs. By this time, the hypodermic syringe and needle were ready (see Chapter 7).

In the early twentieth century, sedative drugs called barbiturates were available. They were mainly prescribed as sleeping pills or to relieve anxiety. One popular example went by the trade name Nembutal. At Abbott Laboratories, American chemists Ernest Henry Volwiler (1893–1992) and Donalee Tabern (1900–74) together spent years researching about 200 drugs similar to Nembutal to discover an anaesthetic to use intravenously. In the 1930s, they found it. Instead of taking twenty minutes to lose consciousness, an injection of Pentothal (a.k.a. thiopentone and sodium thiopental) could send someone to sleep before they could count to twenty.

The Japanese attack on Pearl Harbor in December 1941 immediately dragged the US into the Second World War. It also brought the wide, though not always wise, use of Pentothal. Giving an anaesthetic was often left to the less experienced, especially in wartime. Worse, many of the injured servicemen and women were already in shock before they underwent surgery. Unfortunately, Pentothal made things worse, especially when the drug was used not only to induce anaesthesia, but to keep the casualty asleep for longer procedures. Like many medical students, I was taught that more soldiers died at Pearl Harbor by the misuse of Pentothal than from their injuries. It's probably an exaggeration, but nobody will ever know for sure because records made at the time weren't nearly detailed enough. Another important outcome from Pearl Harbor was improvement in the field of anaesthetics. Still, it's a painfully familiar story of things changing for the better only after a shocking number of deaths.

In the middle of the twentieth century, the use of Pentothal steered away from the strictly medical. In the murky world of spying, the drug got itself a reputation as a truth serum because it was believed to help retrieve repressed memories. Some of the memories recovered may have been fantasy, but that didn't inhibit espionage agencies. Pentothal also found a use in US penitentiaries as one ingredient in a lethal injection. The media played its part in publicizing these uses of Pentothal in films and on TV. Revulsion followed. Protests widened out into the issues of forced interrogations, covert operations, and the death penalty. Eventually, Pentothal fell out of favour.

In the 1980s, a new drug called propofol came onto the market. It wasn't just that Pentothal's reputation was tarnished. Propofol had the benefit of leaving patients feeling far more clear-headed after their anaesthetic.

Anaesthetists began telling people that when they woke up they'd be lucid enough to do the crossword in *The Times* newspaper. That is quite some promise, unless you're already good at cryptic crosswords, but it underlines one of propofol's main benefits, making the drug especially helpful for day-case surgery.

⋙⋘

This is a good place to point out differences in practice and terminology between the US and the UK. An 'anesthetist' in the US means a nurse or someone else who deals with anaesthetics but isn't a doctor. In the UK, however, an 'anaesthetist' is a specialist doctor. It corresponds with the American term 'anesthesiologist', a word that really only came into use in the 1940s, when more doctors became interested in anaesthetics (or should I say 'anesthesiology'?) as a career choice. The speciality has also evolved into the management of intensive-care patients, which needs many of the same skills as looking after someone in the operating theatre.

As for the word 'anaesthesia' itself, it comes from the Greek *anaisthesia*, meaning without sensation. The great American writer and physician Oliver Wendell Holmes, Sr (1809–94) coined the term and suggested it to dentist William Morton in November 1846, a month after Morton's first triumph with ether. Nobody seems to have a copy of the letter in which the word appeared, but there's evidence going back to a publication of 1847 that it really did happen, and that Wendell Holmes spelled 'anaesthesia' the British way.

⋙⋘

One important drug from plants is curare. To be accurate, the word 'curare' refers to a group of similar compounds, originally harvested from the jungle vine *Strychnos toxifera* and other plants. It was used for centuries in South America, mainly in poison-tipped arrows for hunting. Once it reached the bloodstream, the quarry died either because its respiratory muscles were paralyzed, or because it became too weak to run away. Curare doesn't work when taken by mouth. That's good news for the hunter. They can safely eat something or someone killed by a poisoned arrow. Several explorers including Sir Walter Raleigh (1552–1618) brought home their knowledge of various forms of curare, but the drug was barely investigated at the time. Then, not long before the Second World War, interest in curare coincided with new research into how nerves and muscles work.

In the late 1930s, the pharmaceutical company Squibb of New Jersey launched an extract of curare under the name Intocostrin. It was a mix of compounds, the main one being d-tubocurarine. The huge benefit of adding curare to the anaesthetic was that it paralyzed muscle. Without muscle relaxation, it would be difficult to operate in the abdomen, let alone inside the chest. One could achieve this by using high doses of general anaesthetic, at the risk of endangering breathing and the circulation, and delaying recovery. The patient would emerge from surgery, if at all, in very much worse condition than before they went under the knife.

The first reported operation using curare was in January 1942, when the Canadian anaesthesiologist

Harold Griffith (1894–1985) injected a preparation of it into a young man about to have his appendix removed. Thus began the age of muscle relaxants in surgery. That isn't Griffith's only legacy. He realized that care of the patient continued after the final stitch went in. As a result, he set up the first post-op recovery room in Canada. This is now the norm in most parts of the world.

Eventually, ether and chloroform made way for newer gases, like the fluorinated hydrocarbons. To put it simply, these contain fluorine and are derived from ether, but are far more effective as anaesthetics. One of these gases, halothane, came into being in the 1950s thanks to a British chemist called Charles Suckling (1920–2013). Unfortunately, side effects soon reared their head. In 1958, a thirty-nine-year-old woman developed hepatitis that was later recognized as being due to halothane. The hunt for less dangerous anaesthetics was on once again.

Nowadays, isoflurane, desflurane, and sevoflurane are used, although halothane still has a place. Nitrous oxide has also stood the test of time for its pain-killing properties. The patient needs oxygen as well, exactly as Antoine Lavoisier understood over two centuries ago.

The typical anaesthetic workstation today is a world away from the days of a tablecloth soaked in chloroform, or even from Clover's ether inhaler. For one thing, it's all computer-controlled. As well as a supply of gases, a workstation incorporates electronic monitors to check on them, and a host of monitors to keep tabs on the patient's condition. A ventilator is part of the set-up too. There are also disposable syringes and needles for injectable anaesthetics, or for drugs to combat nausea and vomiting.

This complex piece of kit needs electricity to keep it going, so it incorporates a battery as backup. Nothing is ever failsafe, alas, and emergencies can occur. On both sides of the Atlantic, an old adage has it that anaesthetics is 99 per cent boredom and 1 per cent panic, which is just as true as when I first heard it many decades ago. Today's sophisticated machinery still relies on a professional team to deliver the anaesthetic, and to keep the equipment functioning. It's good to know that medically qualified anaesthetists have thorough training, as do the assistants and the technicians who keep the machinery in good order.

Modern anaesthesia began with dentistry, but these days most dental work requires only local numbing, not unconsciousness. Many other procedures, too, can be done while the patient is wide awake, or perhaps lightly sedated.

Techniques for local anaesthesia are often said to go back to the late eighteenth century. However, paintings of devices to numb the limbs were found inside the Egyptian tomb of Saqqara, and that's at least 4,000 years ago. Around 1,000 CE, Anglo-Saxon monks applied cold water or ice to deaden parts of the body before simple surgical procedures. During the Napoleonic Wars, the military surgeon Larrey discovered that amputation was a lot less painful if the casualty's limb was already half frozen, as it often was in Napoleon's retreat from Moscow. Even today, cooling and freezing methods are popular, for instance for piercings.

In the eighteenth century, surgeon James Moore (1762–1860) used much the same technique of nerve compression as the Ancient Egyptians. He studied medicine in Edinburgh and London, then served as a British Army surgeon during the American Revolution. He was a staunch friend of Edward Jenner and a keen advocate of vaccines, but he had many other interests too. He published biographies, and he wrote extensively on the reduction of pain during surgery. There weren't any locally acting drugs at the time – to his knowledge. One of Moore's publications described nerve compression as a way of inducing numbness for operations on a limb. He used a device with adjustable clamps that could be adapted to limbs of most sizes. The distinguished surgeon John Hunter (1728–93), no less, used this exact method for an amputation. Nerve compression was reported as highly successful, but as far as we know, it didn't catch on.

James Moore's arsenal may not have contained locally acting drugs, but they did exist. For over 3,000 years, the native people of the Andes had used coca. This is a South American plant that grows in humid conditions and contains many active components, including cocaine. Peruvians who chewed coca leaves could often work very long hours without stopping to eat or feeling tired.

Coca and cocaine eventually reached Europe in the 1850s, and they soon attracted attention from medics, including two doctors at the Vienna General Hospital. One was a young ophthalmologist by the name of Carl Koller (1857–1944) and the other was Sigmund Freud (1856–1939). On Koller's wish list was a drug to numb the eye for surgery such as procedures for glaucoma. Freud was more intrigued by the use of cocaine to treat morphine addiction. While Freud was at it, he couldn't help noticing a number of other effects, one of them being a boost in libido.

So while Koller pursued his experiments on guinea pigs, Freud left Vienna in great excitement to pursue his fiancée, Martha Bernays. As a result, Koller went down in history as the doctor who first used cocaine for eye surgery. Both he and Freud had researched the drug, but Koller got the credit for its clinical use while Freud got Martha.

Unfortunately, cocaine was highly addictive, which wasn't immediately obvious in the initial enthusiasm for it. In the US, surgeon William Halsted used it to block individual nerves. He also experimented on himself, which was not unusual at the time. Unfortunately, Halsted developed a cocaine addiction. This did not improve when he then tried to treat it with morphine.

Many others took up the practice of local anaesthesia. In Germany in the late 1890s, surgeon August Karl Bier (1861–1949) and his lab assistant August Hildebrandt carried out injections of cocaine into the spine, practising on each other until they were satisfied they could inflict vicious attacks without the victim feeling a thing. To be strictly accurate, it was Bier who hit his assistant's shin with a hammer, put out cigarettes on his thigh, and pummelled his testicles. This proved to both parties that spinal anaesthesia worked. And the method still works today.

Bier also developed regional anaesthesia of a limb. If a tourniquet is in place, an injection of local anaesthetic spreads to the nerves nearby without flooding the circulation. The technique is called Bier's block and is still used today. The drugs themselves, though, have moved on from cocaine. Apart from addiction, its many side effects include giddiness, muscle twitching, a racing pulse, high blood pressure, and even death. More recent compounds are lidocaine (also called lignocaine and Xylocaine) and ropivacaine, which came into use in 1996.

In the very early days, patients were given random compounds in the hope of relieving pain or at least preventing them from running off mid-surgery. Now, anaesthetics is not only more advanced, it's also more patient-centred. In many cases, the dose of anaesthetic is no longer in the doctor's hands. Since the Second World War, women have inhaled so-called gas and air (nitrous oxide and oxygen) during labour, adjusting the amount they breathe to coincide with a contraction. Since the 1980s, it's also become possible for patients to control their own dose of epidural anaesthetic. The concept of letting the patient, where possible, regulate their own pain relief is more logical as well as more caring. After all, it's their pain, not the doctor's.

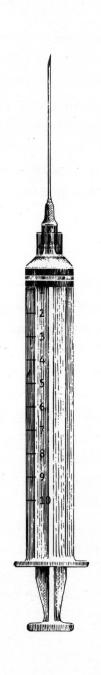

7

The Hypodermic Needle and Syringe: at the Sharp End of Treatment

There's never been a shortage of remedies aimed at making a sick person feel better, but how to get them inside the patient? When the treatment can't be swallowed, sniffed, applied to the skin, or inserted into any pre-existing orifice, physicians look for other ways to deliver it into the body. Efforts to access the bloodstream go back to at least the time of Hippocrates. The methods included placing plant extracts into open wounds and pouring decoctions into specially made incisions.

Syringe-like devices came into use long before needles. The first examples were made from pig bladders, pipes, and quills. Greek physician Galen described impromptu gadgets for applying medicinal salves and ointments. They were also useful for anointing the body with oils, irrigating wounds, and giving enemas.

The word syringe itself comes from the Greek word *syrinx*, meaning pipe or tube. In Greek mythology, Syrinx was an Arcadian nymph of peerless chastity. When Pan pursued her, she escaped into the river. For added protection from him, she asked to be transformed into a reed. But she did not quite avoid Pan's clutches. He sliced up the hollow reeds, made them into his legendary pipes, and has rarely been seen without them since.

Over time, many physicians tried their hand at intravenous infusion (IV). Allegedly, one of the first patients was Pope Innocent VIII (1432–92), who had a stroke in 1492. His doctor tried to bring him round from his coma by transfusing blood directly from three donors. Their chosen technique, according to one popular account, was to cut open the veins of three healthy boys as well as those of the pontiff, stitch them all together, and hope for the best. None of the four participants survived. For a long while after that, other attempts at intravenous infusion met with a similar degree of success.

A lot more science was needed. In about 1650, French mathematician, physicist, inventor, philosopher, and all-round prodigy Blaise Pascal (1623–62) contributed what is now known as Pascal's law or principle. It states that when there is an increase in pressure at any point in a confined fluid, there is an equal increase at every other point in the container. This may sound dull to some, but it is an essential principle governing hydraulic systems, whether it's a medical syringe or the brakes on a car.

British architect Christopher Wren (1632–1723), better known for St Paul's Cathedral in London than for his clinical skills, made use of Pascal's principle to experiment with intravenous injections. In the 1650s, he injected a number of dogs with alcohol, opium, and other substances to see what effect these might have. He did this by cutting into the skin and then into the vein where he inserted a goose quill connected to a pig bladder containing the drug. It's believed that some of the dogs may have survived.

Wren then tried injecting a human being, described as the 'delinquent servant of a foreign ambassador'. Little is known of the man except that he fainted early on in the process. It may have been a ploy to avoid what was coming next. Either way, the experiment was abandoned.

Mid-seventeenth-century England saw further attempts at injection. Needles as such still did not exist, but there was great interest in IV administration, particularly of jalap resin. Jalap was a laxative prepared from the root of a Mexican plant related to morning glory (*Ipomoea*). It was said to be a sovereign remedy for syphilis. Whether or not it solved the problem, jalap gave us the word 'jollop', still used today as a synonym for cathartics and other medicines.

Interest in injection went beyond Britain. Two German doctors in particular gained a reputation for their experiments. Johann Daniel Major (1634–93) was a physician and naturalist, and was a plague doctor in the 1660s (see Chapter 3). Major took injections a step further than Wren and is believed to have been the first person to have successfully injected medicine into a human vein.

Physician Johann Sigismund Elsholtz (1623–88) was a pioneer of hygiene, who gave advice on wholesome food and drink. However, you may find his work on dogs somewhat less wholesome. Using a syringe he'd devised, which he called a 'new clyster', he injected a series of dogs with substances including opium, good Spanish wine, arsenic, and an emetic prepared from *crocus metallorum*. The last two substances turned out to be fatal. Elsholtz also transfused blood from dog to dog, and made some tentative transfusions in humans as well. He suggested that a husband with a 'melancholic nature' could be helped by transfusing blood from his 'vibrant wife'. As far as we know, he didn't put this idea into practice, even though he was convinced it would lead to a more agreeable marriage.

For another couple of centuries, simpler methods of giving medicine appeared safer. Drugs were administered via the skin in the form of ointments and lotions, followed by brisk rubbing. Another tactic to improve absorption was to remove the outer layer of skin with a caustic agent, so that the drug went straight onto the dermis.

In the early nineteenth century, many so-called alkaloid drugs were isolated for the first time from plants. Instead of using crude preparations already in use, physicians now had purer substances such as morphine, colchicine, and atropine. Along with these came methods for giving drugs beneath the skin. However, one of the problems was quantifying the dose of the medicine.

⁂

By and large, getting substances out of the body has been an easier business. In the eleventh century CE, Egyptian ophthalmologist Ammar al-Mawsili (*c.*996–1020 CE) crafted a needle from a hollow glass tube and applied suction to remove his patients' cataracts. As he wrote in his work *Kitāb al-muntakhab fī ilm al-ayn* (The Book of Choice in Ophthalmology), 'with this needle nobody preceded me. I have done many operations with it in Egypt.' Al-Mawsili's ingenious method is still the procedure used today for cataract extractions. Until the thirteenth century, it was also used to extract blood or poison, though not to inject anything.

When it came to extracting blood, nobody did it better than *Hirudo medicinalis*, a.k.a. the medical leech. The use of leeches goes back to Ancient Egypt. A painting in the tomb of eighteenth-dynasty pharaohs (1567–1308 BCE) shows a barber-surgeon applying them to a patient. Documents reveal that leeching was also a remedy in India about 3,300 years ago. Greek and Arab physicians set leeches to work too. Bloodletting was often done in accordance with the humoral therapy, as described by Hippocrates and his followers in the fifth century BCE. This had it that the four humours – blood, phlegm, black bile, and yellow bile – had to be in balance. A disparity in their relative amounts would lead to ill health. If the patient's skin was red from fever or inflammation, there was obviously too much blood. Someone who was strident might also be suffering from excess blood. Bloodletting would rebalance the proportions and restore good health. Whatever was wrong, whether it was skin disease, laryngitis, reproductive problems, and even polio, leeches were a favourite treatment.

Leeches are carnivorous worms that live in fresh water and are hermaphrodites. *Hirudo medicinalis* has two suckers. After piercing the skin, it sucks blood out while injecting anticoagulants. Without these anticoagulants, blood clots would kill the leech. Large adult leeches can take up to two hours to feed, and consume around ten times their body weight in a single meal, or around 5–15 ml (1–3 teaspoons). That's only an approximation of the blood loss, because the patient continues to bleed even after the leech is removed.

Bloodletting with leeches reached its peak in the middle of the nineteenth century. By then, the world was on the cusp of fresh knowledge that was to signal the end of leeching, at least as it was practised then.

Leeches still have a role in the twenty-first century. Research shows that, in addition to anticoagulants, their saliva contains a range of active substances, some of which are antibacterial. Since around 1980, plastic surgery units the world over have used leeches to reduce venous congestion and increase the viability of skin flaps and replanted digits. As for the leeches, they can live for up to a year between feeds. But they don't. The risk of bloodborne disease means that leeches aren't reused for other patients. Once their job is done, they are dunked in 70 per cent alcohol, which promptly kills them.

As far as administering therapy went, all the methods were a bit hit and miss – until, that is, Irish physician Francis Rynd (1801–61) came along. Rynd had been an unruly medical student who preferred hunting and horse riding to working on the wards. After graduating, he became a sought-after doctor who hobnobbed with Dublin nobility. He dressed fashionably and was popular with the ladies, though less so with his peers. Today he is best remembered for fashioning a thin tube from a strip of steel. He drew the tube through ever narrower holes to reduce the bore. One end of the tube was then bevelled and ground. Rynd added a fitting at the other end and set to work.

Fifty-nine-year-old Margaret Cox had endured the pain of neuralgia for six years. She had already sought relief by drinking a solution of morphine. On 3 June 1844, Rynd mixed a preparation of fifteen grains of acetate of morphia (about 970 mg) in one drachm of creosote (about 3.5 ml). Using his new needle, he made four separate punctures on his patient's face and administered the drug along the supra-orbital, temporal, malar, and buccal nerves. It seemed to work. Margaret Cox was back on top form.

Today, we know that it was the solvent that did the trick, not the generous dose of morpine. Creosote is toxic to nerves and must have blocked transmission of pain signals. Even so, Rynd's little invention proved useful to many. At one point, Florence Nightingale (1820–1910) herself had a similar treatment. Nothing, she declared, was better for the pain of her illness than this curious little procedure of placing opium under the skin. Rynd made a fortune from his practice, but then lost a large amount of it in imprudent investments.

In 1861, he wrote a paper describing his subcutaneous injection technique. That same year, he died a death as dramatic as his life had been. His carriage knocked a woman down in the street. When he went to check that she was unharmed, a group of men attacked the carriage. There was a skirmish and Rynd went in pursuit of the men. Witnesses said they saw him slump over the reins as his horse bolted. He died on the way to hospital, possibly from a heart attack.

∞

With Rynd's needle, the drug flowed into the body under gravity. It was Frenchman Charles Pravaz who invented a plunger syringe for injections. Few people have heard of Charles Gabriel Pravaz (1791–1853). Even fewer can say whether he was a vet or an orthopaedic surgeon. He may have been both. It's known that he treated animals and that he had an interest in applying his methods to humans.

In 1853, Pravaz was experimenting with injections under the skin of sheep. He hoped to inject coagulant into an aneurysm, a technique used today by radiologists. But Pravaz needed better tools for the job. He took Rynd's type of needle, measuring 3 cm (1 in) long and 5 mm (⅛ in) in diameter, and added a screw-operated syringe specially made by notable instrument makers Établissements Charrière (see Chapter 2, page 42). It was a precision-crafted syringe containing just 1 ml. Made entirely of silver, its barrel concealed the contents so it must have been hard to control the amount of drug injected.

Unlike Rynd, Pravaz died before publishing. But another French practitioner championed his innovation.

Jules Béhier (1813–76) was linked with the most prestigious hospitals in Paris, including the Hôpital Pitié and the Hôtel-Dieu. He used his clout to make Pravaz's work known throughout Europe, and to introduce sclerotherapy injections as a treatment for varicose veins. Not all Béhier's therapies came in the form of injections. He also tried to popularize cold water treatment for typhoid and alcoholic drinks for pneumonia, both allegedly English remedies.

Pravaz's syringe was only the start. Injection therapy had a long way to go and obstacles to overcome, some of them unknown at the time, like the danger of infection. As it turned out, 1853 was a good year for the hypodermic syringe. The person most often linked with its invention is not Pravaz, but physician Alexander Wood (1817–84). Inspired by fellow Scotsman James Young Simpson's work with anaesthesia (see Chapter 6, page 123), Wood set out to find ways of relieving localized pain.

In 1853, Wood took Rynd's earlier device of a fine-bore needle and added a plunger syringe. His syringe was all glass, so one could see and control the amount of drug injected – a refinement that was perhaps superfluous at the time, since doctors weren't sure of the right dose. Wood's first patient was an eighty-year-old woman with troublesome neuralgia in her shoulder. He injected the area of pain with morphine dissolved in sherry. His patient slept for ten hours thereafter, which annoyed Wood. On the other hand, her pain had vanished, so both of them were pleased with the end result. Wood had thus successfully used the world's first plunger-operated hypodermic syringe.

The synchronicity may seem odd, but there's no evidence that Wood and Pravaz even knew of each other. Quite simply, the hypodermic was an idea whose time had come. But why do so few people today credit Pravaz? Perhaps it's because he worked with sheep rather than humans. Or perhaps because he died before writing up his work, in a fateful illustration of the dictum to publish or perish.

Wood was also a respected professional whose stature far exceeded Pravaz's. Wood became President of the Royal College of Physicians of Edinburgh. He used his influence to campaign for the registration of births and marriages, led the way for sanitary reform, and pressed for help for the unemployed. He supported extramural education in Edinburgh, which, among other things, eventually helped women study medicine. Wood also had strong views about medicine and how it should be practised. He believed in a properly licensed group of medical practitioners. A scientist at heart, he spoke up against unorthodox treatments such as homeopathy.

His device was advertised as 'Dr Alexander Wood's narcotic injection syringe'. He and his treatment soon became popular. When Wood died, he left his wife, Rebecca, and his hypodermic syringe, with a design not so different from that used today. What he didn't leave behind was the word 'hypodermic'. Wood always called his injections 'subcutaneous'.

The term 'hypodermic' was coined in 1858 by a much younger doctor from London. Charles Hunter (1835–78) was a mere house surgeon at St George's Hospital when he began to research methods of pain relief. Before long, Hunter's work and opinions had antagonized Wood.

According to Wood, pain-killing injections only worked locally, so they had to be made directly into the painful area. Hunter, however, claimed that they could be given anywhere because their effect was more widespread. He knew it for a fact. On one occasion, when his patient had an abscess over the area of pain, Hunter had been forced to choose a different injection site. Even so, the patient obtained relief from the treatment. Hunter had then tested it out on animals. It was no fluke.

Wood may have realized that the young whippersnapper from London had a point. When Wood injected morphine along a nerve, he often found that the patient became very drowsy, just as his first patient with neuralgia had, suggesting that at least some of the drug had reached the brain. Nonetheless, the disagreement with Hunter continued and there was a drawn-out correspondence in the *Medical Times and Gazette*. Of course, Hunter responded with his belief in the general effect of injected morphine. In 1865 he published his results and addressed various medical society meetings. In 1867, the Medical and Chirurgical Society of London decided that a scientific committee had to settle the debate. The committee examined the evidence and endorsed Hunter.

Hunter died at the age of forty-three after a short illness. His early death coupled with Wood's status means that Charles Hunter is not as well known today as he might have been. Once again, the more eminent man's name prevailed. But Hunter did give us the word 'hypodermic'. It comes from the Greek words *hypo* (meaning under) and *derma* (meaning skin). He called it *ipodermic* to begin with, but soon revised it to the version we know today.

∝⚬

The use of the hypodermic needle and syringe relied on a better understanding of the circulation. For that, we have to thank English physician William Harvey (1578–1657). Harvey gained his first degree from Gonville and Caius College, Cambridge, which was co-founded by John Caius (1510–73), a proponent of dissection. This art shaped Harvey's work. After studying medicine in Padua, Harvey became physician extraordinary to King James I.

In Harvey's day, doctors believed that the lungs acted as bellows to keep blood moving. Another misconception of the time was that blood was constantly generated from food, and was then used up by the tissues and organs of the body. Harvey disproved all that. Most of his research centred on how blood flowed around the human body, although he dissected a fair few animals to reach that point. In 1628, he published his renowned *Exercitatio Anatomica de Motu Cordis et Sanguinis in Animalibus* (An Anatomical Disputation of the Movement of the Heart and Blood in Animals), often known as *De Motu Cordis*. It was translated from Latin to English in around 1648, when Harvey was seventy years old. It took much longer than that for his ideas to be accepted because they contradicted received wisdom. The conviction persisted that any injected medicine only exerted a local effect and could not spread to the rest of the body, and, as we've seen, even the eminent Alexander Wood refused to take it on board two centuries later.

Harvey showed that heart muscle contraction (a phase called 'systole') served to pump out the blood. Blood was not consumed. It returned to the heart, with valves in the veins allowing only one-way flow. He demonstrated that blood flowed in two separate circuits, the systemic circulation and the pulmonary circulation. Less well supported by evidence was Harvey's enduring belief in witches. According to him, most women had the potential to wreak havoc, and Europeans had no idea how to keep them in check.

Whomever you prefer to credit, the hypodermic needle and syringe were finally here. They soon became essential, either for removing fluids from the body or for administering substances. Nowadays we have injections of all types, including intravenous, intramuscular, subcutaneous, and even injections into the spine, along with all the benefits of anaesthesia, vaccinations, chemotherapy, blood tests, and blood transfusion. This little object is indispensable to modern medicine.

While the modern syringe exists in various forms, almost all are versions of the same concept. The all-glass Lüer syringe goes back to 1894 and Parisian instrument maker Hermann Wülfing-Lüer (1836–1910). Born Hermann Wülfing, he was originally from Germany. His firm was responsible for the unique graduated all-glass hypodermic syringe, although it's unclear exactly who designed it. It could have been one of his engineers. Then again, it may have been his wife, Jeanne Amélie Lüer (1842–1909). The daughter of surgical instrument maker Amatus Lüer, she worked on the creative side of the company while her husband managed the business. The Lüer syringe resisted heat, so it allowed steam sterilizing at 120°C (248°F). Best of all, it had a conical tip with a 6 per cent taper, which made for rapid leak-free connecting. The Lüer fitting is still in use today.

Production expanded across the Atlantic. In 1897, businessmen Maxwell W. Becton (1868–1951) and Fairleigh S. Dickinson (1866–1948), both from North Carolina, formed an import company named BD or Becton-Dickinson. In 1898, they acquired a half-interest in the patent rights to the all-glass syringes developed by Wülfing-Lüer and started selling them for $2.50 apiece.

◦⚬⚬◦

The turn of the century was a time of huge innovation, when patents rapidly followed one another. In 1899, New Yorker Letitia Mumford Geer (1852–1935) submitted a patent for a one-handed syringe design. As a nurse, she had noticed that doctors sometimes needed help to use a syringe. Her version incorporated a U-shaped handle, so, even at extreme positions of the plunger, one hand could control both the plunger and the cylinder. As well as founding the Geer Manufacturing Company to develop her design, she invented the nasal speculum and a surgical retractor. She also became an activist and suffragist.

Back in East Rutherford, New Jersey, BD set up its production plant to manufacture hypodermic needles, syringes, and thermometers, all of which the company still makes today. Around 1930, BD launched its Yale Luer-Lok Syringe, designed by Dickinson. Instead of being tapered, the tip was threaded for a more secure attachment to a needle.

Well into the 1950s, hypodermic syringes were re-usable, as were needles. These glass syringes were expensive and fragile, and it was a palaver to sterilize them between patients. To prevent cracking, nurses had to wrap them in cotton cloth before exposing them to heat. If there was no autoclave to provide steam heat under pressure, boiled water was the next best thing. Sometimes, the plunger would stick, and another device was needed to separate it from the barrel. As for the needles, they were less fragile but they eventually became blunt through use.

Disposable syringes were heaven-sent to those at the sharp end of healthcare. But, for a long time, disposables were also made of glass. BD first produced their HYPAK syringe on a large scale in 1954, just in time for the rollout of the polio vaccine created by Jonas Salk (1914–95). In 1955, Roehr Products of Connecticut launched a plastic disposable syringe. The Monoject sold for 5 US cents each, but a lot of doctors still thought it was cheaper to sterilize and reuse glass syringes.

American neuropsychiatrist Albert Weiner should perhaps take some credit for the demise of the reusable syringe. Weiner (dates unknown) was both an osteopath and a psychiatrist. In his busy New Jersey practice, he gave patients muscle relaxants for ECT at such a rate that he was dubbed the world's fastest psychiatrist. In 1960, a record number of his patients developed the blood-borne infection viral hepatitis. Experts declared this could not be chance. Patients testified that they had seen blood on syringes. It all suggested that sterilization of the equipment had not been ideal. The market for disposable syringes boomed.

When it comes to vaccinating, a prefilled disposable syringe is even more convenient. Colin Murdoch (1929–2008) came up with the first one in 1956, when he was twenty-seven. He was a New Zealand veterinarian and pharmacist looking for an easier way to vaccinate animals. He also invented the tranquillizer gun and the world's first childproof medicine bottle cap. It's said that his nights were filled with vivid dreams of new devices, and he would leap out of bed to set it all down on paper. During his lifetime, Murdoch held some forty-six patents, and many benefited from his inventions. This includes some companies that violated his patents. Murdoch never sued.

Today's syringes are almost all plastic disposables. Worldwide, the standard is the Luer-tipped syringe. A need for standardization became painfully clear at an air show in 1988. Three Italian aircraft collided mid-air at USAF Ramstein in West Germany, and then fell to the ground in flames. There may have been communication problems between the US military and the German paramedics. There was definitely incompatibility between their resuscitation equipment. Their IV catheters used different types of connectors, which delayed treatment of many of the casualties. International standards for syringes came in a few years later.

Luer fittings are now king, at least for hypodermic needles and those intended for blood vessels. There are specific non-Luer connectors for other uses. An intentional mismatch is a good way to prevent errors. If the same connector is used for every purpose, there's the risk of a drug meant for IV use ending up in a spinal injection instead, with fatal results.

As I mentioned earlier in this chapter, the very first blood transfusion was believed to have been carried out on Pope Innocent VIII with the help of some imaginative suturing. However, as the distinguished surgeon and historian Geoffrey Keynes (1887–1982) later pointed out, this so-called transfusion was no more than a draught taken by mouth. It had been prepared from the blood of three healthy boys who then died soon after their donation.

Nobody is quite sure when blood transfusion began. In the seventeenth century in both Paris and London, there were many attempts at transfusing animal blood into humans, and almost as many failures. The whole enterprise was somewhat haphazard. In 1901, however, Austrian immunologist Karl Landsteiner (1868–1943) and his colleagues discovered three ABO blood groups. This made transfusion more scientific, and more successful.

Initially, transfusions had to take place directly from donor to recipient because clotting was a problem. Use of sodium citrate as an anticoagulant in 1914 opened up new possibilities. The First World War brought advances in transfusion, too, thanks to the altruism of donors and the ingenuity of military medics. But there were organizational hurdles. Refrigerating citrated blood meant it could be stored for two to three days. Eventually, adding glucose enabled storage for two to three weeks. Blood banking had arrived.

In 1937, Landsteiner and Alexander Solomon Wiener (1907–76) made another leap forward when they discovered the Rhesus blood group system. This further improved transfusion and also had a positive impact on the pregnancies of Rhesus-negative women.

Blood transfusion became far more feasible towards the Second World War. US surgeon and researcher Charles R. Drew (1904–50) translated test-tube procedures into a technique for mass-producing plasma from whole blood. Plasma is a clear yellow fluid that is rich in protein but does not contain blood cells. During the war, transfusion of plasma instead of red blood cells proved vital because it could restore lost blood volume and provide coagulation factors at the same time. Drew became medical director of the Blood for Britain project, which provided US blood and plasma to British soldiers and civilians. One of the very few African-Americans in his field, he protested against the practice of racially segregating blood donation, which had no scientific basis and was wholly racist. Drew died at the age of forty-five in a car accident. After operating through the night, the exhausted Drew lost control of his car the next morning.

The hypodermic also transformed the outlook of diabetes. Insulin was discovered in 1921, but it had to be injected. The advent of insulin treatment in the early 1920s gave a huge boost to the market for syringes. More importantly, insulin injections changed lives. Until then, fasting was the main treatment, which killed some patients.

Could people with diabetes inject their own insulin? Many doubted that patients would have the intellect to do so. It might also make them less dependent on health professionals. A shocking suggestion.

One American doctor had the answer. Massachusetts physician Elliott Proctor Joslin (1869–1962) was inspired by his aunt's diabetes, and then his mother's. He went on to research it for the rest of his life, and became the country's first diabetologist. Joslin's views were astonishing at the time. According to him, patients could and should be charged with managing their own diabetes. As early as 1923, Joslin declared that they needed no more than a week to learn how to handle their diet and their insulin.

He was proved right, and this is now the model for diabetes care. Few patients had difficulties, although it was sometimes a challenge to work out the dose of insulin. Some preparations came in 20 U/ml, others twice or four times that. It wasn't until the early 1980s that so-called U-100 became the norm, where each ml of an insulin preparation contains 100 units of insulin. The standard syringe now has units and marks that correspond.

Even more convenient is a syringe with a needle permanently attached to it. In 1981, Scottish physician John Ireland (1933–88) came up with the idea of the insulin pen – the Penject – and the company Novo Nordisk made the pen a commercial reality. Since then, Novo Nordisk and other makers have ensured that few people have to use an old-style syringe for their insulin.

It seems curious there was such resistance to people with diabetes handling their own insulin, when so many other people were already abusing drugs by self-injection. Not everything about the hypodermic has been positive, and it wasn't long after its development that drug abuse emerged. To be strictly accurate, it was there already. Opiates were commonplace in Victorian Britain. Morphine could be taken in tablet form, or mixed with alcohol to make laudanum, a libation much enjoyed by the writer Thomas De Quincey (1785–1859), whose 1812 memoir *Confessions of an English Opium-Eater* chronicles his dependence. Whatever the complaint, whether it was a headache or a stomach ulcer, many thought morphine was the answer. Before long, opium eaters turned into opium injectors. Some users injected themselves daily, especially if they were affluent women with chronic conditions like neuralgia or insomnia. By 1875, there were even mini-syringes that could be carried about on a key chain to make self-injection more convenient. Today, auto-injectors filled with epinephrine (adrenaline) are life-saving for those with anaphylaxis and other severe allergies.

Intravenous drug abuse is a more recent phenomenon. It's said to have existed in China in the early twentieth century, along with needle sharing. It was certainly recorded in the 1920s in the US and in Egypt, and it may have caused malaria outbreaks between 1929 and 1937. Drug abuse is ever-present, and with it the risk of infection, especially with blood-borne diseases such as hepatitis and human immunodeficiency virus (HIV). Users tend to reuse their equipment unless they have access to fresh supplies. One way of ensuring syringes really are single-use is to choose versions like the K1 auto-disable syringe, invented in the late 1990s. Once the plunger on the K1 is depressed, it's impossible to pull it up again.

Almost any injection has the potential to introduce pathogens from the skin into the body. But is it necessary to disinfect the skin before an injection or blood test? That depends on the site of the puncture, the gauge of the needle, and the person's health. On the whole, microorganisms on the skin are too few to cause infection from a puncture with a very fine needle like a 25 or 27 gauge. For most insulin injections, then, swabbing the skin is superfluous, especially since insulin preparations contain phenol, which is a disinfectant.

Having a blood test is another matter. The needle is a little wider, and the cubital fossa (the area in front of the elbow) is moist enough to encourage bacteria. Cleaning the skin is in order when taking blood for donation, too. For immunizations, though, most vaccinators agree that only visibly dirty skin merits cleaning.

Needles have become sharper and less painful since 1844 when Francis Rynd injected the first patient. Even so, many people today go out of their way to avoid a hypodermic. It's thought that some 10 per cent of the population may have trypanophobia. Needle phobia is even more common in children and young adults. One solution is anaesthetic cream applied ahead of time. Other techniques include distraction, hypnosis, graded exposure to needles, and cognitive behavioural therapy (CBT). Needle phobia may sound trivial to those who don't have it, but it can have serious consequences, such as avoidance of vaccinations, blood tests, and even life-saving treatments. People who fear needles are more likely to become seriously ill as a result of avoiding medical help for a seemingly minor condition that evolves into a severe illness. Unfortunately, a sizeable US study from 2022 found that many with needle phobia did not find the medical profession helpful in dealing with their problem.

Wouldn't it be grand to do away with needles, at least for those who fear them? In 2013, US engineer Mark Prausnitz (b. 1966) launched his Microneedle, a drug delivery system that uses 400 silicon-based needles too fine to stimulate pain receptors. It looks somewhat like a nicotine patch and can administer medicines or vaccines into the body. Microelectronics inside the device regulate dosage of the drug. From an era before the hypodermic, we could now be moving to a future beyond it.

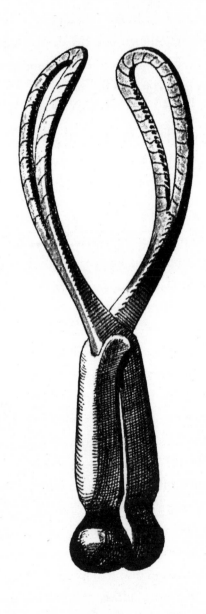

8

Obstetric Forceps: Modern Methods for Birthing Babies

∽⊱⊰∾

The era of obstetric forceps arrived in the early seventeenth century, accompanied by secrecy and subterfuge. The tale is something of a saga featuring the Chamberlens, an enterprising family descended from French Huguenot Guillaume Chamberlen.

Using instruments to aid delivery has a much longer history. Hindu documents describe instrumental vaginal births as far back as the sixth century BCE. Hippocratic writings also refer to instrumental delivery between 500 BCE and 500 CE. The Muslim philosopher and physician Avicenna (980–1037 CE) probably used forceps too. However, the crucial difference is that, in centuries past, they were used only to remove a dead fetus after many days of labour. Whether the operator used surgical tools or kitchen utensils to penetrate the fetal skull, the aim was to save the mother's life, and in some cases also to baptize the dead baby.

It was therefore close to miraculous when the Chamberlen family developed forceps delivery to help both parties survive labour. Exactly what their forceps were and how they did it remained strictly secret for about 100 years. The hint at miracle-working did not hurt their reputation during that time.

This story begins in sixteenth-century France when Queen Catherine de Medici (1519–89) banned Protestant physicians. As a result, the Huguenot doctor Guillaume (William) Chamberlen (*c.*1540–96) fled to England in 1569 with his wife Geneviève and their children, including two sons, Peter Chamberlen the Elder (*c.*1560–1631) and Peter Chamberlen the Younger (1572–1626). It's a little curious to have named both boys Peter, though they did ease the confusion by calling the elder one Pierre.

Nobody seems sure which Chamberlen invented forceps, but it's likely to have been Peter the Elder when, at the very start of the seventeenth century, he was appointed Royal Surgeon and cared for Queen Henrietta Maria, wife of Charles I, during her miscarriage. Medics of the period often protected their methods to prevent others from profiting from them, but the Chamberlens were unusually thorough in their efforts at concealment. They added a dash of theatre by carrying their instruments in an ornate gilded chest so large that it needed two people to lift it. Once in the birth chamber, the chest was opened only when the labouring woman had been blindfolded. Only the Chamberlens were in attendance during the delivery. The family therefore managed to keep their forceps to themselves for a century.

We now know that the Chamberlens tweaked their instrument during this time. At first, the forceps were tricky to manoeuvre, so they replaced the original riveted joint with a pin that worked as a pivot. They eventually decided that a tape to hold the blades together was even better. The forceps had a curve to cradle the infant's head and were open-work to provide a good grip and reduce compression.

Their instruments eventually saw the light of day in 1813 when they were discovered under the floorboards of the attic in their old home, Woodham Mortimer Hall in Essex. Ann Chamberlen, wife of Peter the Third, had for some reason stowed them there. Peter the Third (1601–83) was the eldest son of Peter the Younger and lectured in anatomy. He had a son called Hugh Chamberlen (1630–1720), who came to be known as Hugh the Elder. His two other sons, Paul and John, were man-midwives. The family had an eye for lucrative opportunities but sometimes got it wrong. Paul was involved in what was known as the 'anodyne necklace scandal', which broke in 1715. It was a time of high infant mortality, and there was a profusion of nostrums containing herbs that allegedly protected children against convulsions, teething, rickets, consumption, and anything else believed to endanger health. The so-called anodyne necklace was a particular amulet reputed to have these special powers and then some, and its popularity was almost all Paul Chamberlen's doing. He might not have invented the necklace, but he endorsed it, and people were only too ready to believe in it. He and the necklace were eventually shown to be complete frauds.

As for Hugh the Elder, he was a successful physician but had lost a small fortune in get-rich-quick schemes.

Needing money, he tried to sell the family's trade secret. In 1670, he travelled to France and approached two prominent medical men, François Mauriceau (1637–1709) and Jules (a.k.a. Julien) Clément (1649–1728).

Mauriceau was a surgeon and man-midwife or *accoucheur*, while Clément was the royal *accoucheur*. Hugh the Elder tried to sell Clément his instrument for 10,000 crowns, but Mauriceau wanted a demonstration first. To prove himself and his instrument, Hugh had to deliver a woman who had already been in labour for eight days. She also happened to be thirty-eight years old with dwarfism and a deformed pelvis, so it was quite a test. Hugh the Elder agreed to the conditions and spent the next three hours locked in the lying-in room with the woman. The baby perished, the mother died of a ruptured uterus, and the deal was off. Nonetheless, Hugh's trip yielded other rewards. He managed to get a copy of Mauriceau's recently published textbook *Des maladies des femmes grosses*. Once he'd translated it and published it in 1673 as *The Accomplisht Midwife*, it became required reading on midwifery.

In seventeenth-century France, *accoucheurs* were very much à la mode, thanks to Louis XIV, who appointed them for his many pregnant mistresses. As *accoucheur* to the Sun King's women, Clément was celebrated as much for his discretion as for his clinical expertise. He attended several other noble but clandestine births. At home and abroad, the aristocracy clamoured for his skills. Françoise-Athénaïs de Rochechouart-Mortemart, better known as Madame de Montespan (1640–1707) was the chief royal mistress to Louis XIV. When Clément attended in 1669 to deliver the first of the seven children she had by the king, he was led blindfolded into her quarters to make sure he didn't recognize her. As the tale goes, the king was so delighted at the baby girl's birth that he himself served Clément a glass of wine afterwards.

The role of men in the labour room was on the rise, and with that came improved obstetric forceps from the early 1700s onwards. The French developed a pair of forceps with a joint designed for easier insertion and stabilizing once they were placed around the fetal head. In Paris, André Levret (1703–80) was one of the most illustrious obstetricians. Initially trained in surgery, he moved into obstetrics and eventually became royal *accoucheur*. He wrote what was possibly the first treatise on female anatomy. From his studies, he concluded that forceps needed not only a curve for the baby's head but also a pelvic curve to match the anatomy of the mother. This was a major improvement. That and his writings made him well known in France and abroad. He was also known for his expertise in breech births and caesarean section.

He and other men did more than come up with new tools. They changed how parturition was managed. Until then, the birthing chamber had been women-only. Although each country had its own customs, it was the general view that only women had insight into the wonder of birth and all that came with it. Midwives did not rely on scholarly tomes. They learned hands-on from other midwives how to deliver babies. They had skills in breech as well as normal births. They also cared for women antenatally and postnatally, and they often educated them on contraception, child health, and probably much more. There was no legal requirement to have midwives at a birth, but women liked and trusted them, and that assured their popularity and their survival.

Midwives became sidelined once men played a more important role. But what to call these men? The English word 'midwife' comes from 'with woman' (the woman being the one in labour). In France, the term for 'midwife' was *sage-femme*, meaning a wise woman, with the *femme* part referring to the practitioner. A man who assumed a role in childbirth was dubbed *accoucheur*. In Britain, the term 'man-midwife' seemed insufficiently lofty, and the word 'obstetrician' had yet to catch on. As a result, many, even the British, favoured the French term *accoucheur*.

In Britain, two main groups of men practised midwifery. First, there were some eminent physicians in London and other cities, like Thomas Denman (1733–1815) and William Osborne (1736–1808), who became the first manmidwives recognized by the Royal College of Physicians at the end of the eighteenth century. Then there were surgeon-apothecaries who practised surgery, midwifery, and general medicine. These became general practitioners in the nineteenth century. Until the mid-twentieth century in Britain, they played a central role in labour alongside midwives.

The midwifery specialists or *accoucheurs* wrote widely. Thomas Denman penned a volume of aphorisms on the use of forceps. Medical students would carry a copy of this slim hardback in their coat pockets. Very few copies exist today, probably because they were so well thumbed.

When the Chamberlens found a hiding place beneath the floorboards of Woodham Mortimer Hall, they left behind not one but three obstetric instruments. Along with the forceps, there were also the fillet and the vectis. Thomas Denman first wrote about the vectis in 1783. Part lever, part spoon, the vectis resembled half a pair of forceps and was almost certainly a Chamberlen family invention. Although challenging to use and potentially dangerous with it, the vectis could, with luck, help lever out the baby in some cases when labour was obstructed.

By contrast, the fillet was already known to Avicenna. It was a simple noose of horsehair or leather mounted on a stick. The practitioner would loop it over the baby's chin and manoeuvre the head into a better position before pulling it out. Both instruments must have been lethal, especially in inexperienced hands. Over time, teaching methods changed, and students more often learned in large groups rather than one-to-one as apprentices, which may have contributed to the decline of the vectis in particular. It disappeared from use as well as from most museums. The fillet also all but dropped out of the history books.

The forceps flourished and consolidated the role and reputation of obstetricians. The Midwives Act 1902 established the Central Midwives Board and brought in a more formal delineation of roles. Rules for midwifery practice followed in 1907. While midwives remained responsible for normal labour, the new statutes demanded that they call a doctor to assist with any birth that was not normal. Infraction would lead to removal from the midwives' register.

Just as the Chamberlens had modified and updated their forceps, the new men-midwives also revised the design over the years. William Smellie (1697–1763) came from a Scottish family of modest means. He first worked as an apothecary with a sideline as a draper. As a man-midwife, he aimed to make his speciality more scientific, and went on to give his name to many advances in obstetrics. He believed that only some 10 per cent of births needed forceps. Nonetheless he saw the need for an improved pair of forceps with a pelvic curve and a lock at the pivot point. Each forceps blade was covered in leather to made it noiseless. The forceps could therefore be deployed without the woman or her attendant realizing it. In breech deliveries, Smellie was the first to use forceps on the aftercoming head. He is also believed to have been the first to rotate the head with forceps.

Smellie produced a life-sized model of a pregnant woman for teaching. He kept it in his own home and called it his 'machine'. Leather-covered, it included ligaments, muscles, and skin, all in artificial materials. A cloth doll played the role of fetus. It was said to be more realistic than previous manikins, and no wonder. At least one of his 'machines' wore clothes, stockings, and shoes, all with the aim of educating his students.

Alongside this work, Smellie published his *Treatise on the Theory and Practice of Midwifery*, as well as sets of anatomical tables and illustrations of the pregnant female. Both he and his former pupil William Hunter were the leading obstetric teachers of their day. The elder brother of the celebrated surgeon and collector John Hunter (1728–93), William was a Scottish physician and anatomist. He and Smellie were popular teachers who brought obstetrics to life with detailed drawings to accompany hands-on experience. Less affluent patients were in luck. Smellie offered them free midwifery services if they permitted students to witness a birth. The Father of British Midwifery, as he is sometimes called, died poor but left behind many improvements in obstetrics as well as a dynasty of doctors that includes some prominent members even today.

Wooden-handled forceps slowly gave way to metal, as the instrument also evolved in other ways. One of the finest innovators ever was another Scotsman, the obstetrician Sir James Young Simpson (1811–70). The son of a baker, he was born in West Lothian as James Simpson. The middle name Young has obscure origins but it was definitely a later adoption. Although his family was humble, Simpson was the seventh son, so locals were convinced he was destined for greatness. They were right. Simpson went on to make his mark in both obstetrics and anaesthetics. At school he was an assiduous student and interested in everything around him. He studied at Edinburgh for an arts degree and began his medical studies later, opting for additional classes such as those led by the redoubtable surgeon Robert Liston.

Simpson was by all accounts a character. Usually depicted with unkempt hair and a scruffy beard, he had an impressive intellect and often brimmed with ideas on a range of topics from archaeology to hermaphrodites, which at the time were a taboo subject. When he practised as a country surgeon, midwifery was a large part of his work. From then on, he set his heart on becoming an obstetrician, but he also believed that midwives played a valuable role, even in hospitals. He worked at Edinburgh Royal Dispensary for the Poor and continued with pro bono work in his later life.

Depression set Simpson back repeatedly, though in between episodes he showed prodigious energy. At twenty-four, he was elected president of the Royal Medical Society of Edinburgh. A believer in the rigour of science, he refuted the principles of homeopathy and rejected the literal interpretation of the book of Genesis. He gave a paper entitled *Pathological Observations on the Diseases of the Placenta*. A keen observer, he spotted a link between protein in the urine and the potentially lethal pregnancy complication eclampsia. He recommended monitoring the baby's heart rate, and was one of the first to point out that slowing of the heart rate often came before fetal death. When he spoke in his graduation address in 1832 on the future of medicine, he predicted ways of seeing inside the body with the use of electricity. This was a time when X-rays were still some sixty years in the future.

Simpson's work made Edinburgh a centre of obstetric excellence. We can thank him for three advances in particular. Anaesthesia for childbirth followed on from his work with ether (see Chapter 6, page 123). Just a few months after Morton demonstrated ether in Boston, Simpson used it for a labouring woman with a severely narrow pelvis. The Bible, along with many doctors, may have disapproved of pain-free labour, but Simpson believed that women deserved it.

His name is also closely linked with chloroform. It's a moot point as to whether he discovered the properties of the drug, but he did play a role in deploying it. According to one myth, described in Simpson's biography by his daughter Eve, the mother of the first infant delivered under chloroform named her child 'Anaesthesia'. In reality, the baby was christened Wilhelmina. 'Anaesthesia' was probably Simpson's nickname for her.

The second notable innovation to Simpson's name was his improved design for obstetric forceps, still known today as Simpson's forceps. They had a long curve for the baby's head, ideal when it had already been elongated by time spent in the birth canal.

Simpson also fashioned a suction cup with a piston at its narrow end. He called it his 'air tractor' and thought it might prove useful to help pull out a baby's head. The cup was covered in leather and greased with lard. Although Simpson showed it to colleagues, the method didn't catch on until the ventouse was invented more than 100 years later.

All in all, Simpson was a remarkable doctor who seems to have given more thought than many others to a woman's perspective of labour. Just before he died, he also took up the cause of women in medicine by persuading the powers that be to permit Sophia Jex-Blake (1840–1912) to study medicine. When Simpson died, 30,000 people are said to have lined the streets of the funeral route. There is a statue to him in Princes Street, Edinburgh, as well as a bust in a niche at Westminster Abbey in London.

Another instrument came in around 1867. The Neville Barnes forceps was the brainchild of obstetricians Robert Barnes and William Neville. A busy London doctor, Barnes (1817–1907) worked at several large London hospitals and wrote widely on women's health. He showed his forceps to a meeting of the Obstetrical Society of London in 1867. The forceps were long and the blades were also elongated so as to grasp the moulded fetal head at or above the brim of the pelvis, and hopefully to avoid the need for a caesarean. Barnes also determined the best angle at which to pull.

A little later, William Neville devised his axis-traction handle, which could be attached to most conventional forceps. Neville (1855–1904) was an obstetrician at the Coombe Lying-in Hospital, Dublin, when he designed his apparatus. Ill health, probably TB, soon made him leave obstetrics and turn to pathology. He died before he was fifty.

As anaesthetics became more effective, more interventions became feasible. Instruments multiplied to fill various needs. There are many styles of obstetric forceps, so the rundown here is nothing near a complete list. Further innovations lay in store in the early twentieth century. Norwegian obstetrician Christian Kjelland (1871–1941) came up with forceps that were especially useful for rotating the baby's head into a better position. His forceps were straight, with a head curve only. A pelvic curve would have seriously injured the woman when the forceps were rotated. Kjelland forceps also had a sliding lock mechanism which was useful if the baby's head was tilted to one side.

Kjelland began working with his new instrument in 1908, and it was soon used worldwide. Back home, however, his boss Professor Kristian Brandt (1859–1932) was less impressed. He continued to use Simpson's forceps and didn't even mention Kjelland's in his book on obstetrics. It was as if they had never existed. As a result, his assistant's innovation failed to catch on in Norway.

The early twentieth century also saw in Wrigley's forceps, a short instrument designed by the British obstetrician Arthur Joseph Wrigley (1902–83). Unlike Kjelland, he disliked applying forceps when the head was high up in the pelvis, so he designed a small, lightweight version that was easy to use. As the story goes, a storeman at St Thomas' Hospital, London, was tidying away surgical clutter in the basement when he came across an old pair of short forceps somewhat like Smellie's two centuries earlier. Joe Wrigley, as he was known, was of a practical bent and immediately spotted their potential. He sent them off to instrument makers Allen & Hanbury's, asking them to add a pelvic curve and a short handle. The end result was the Wrigley forceps, weighing just 285 g (10 oz).

Wrigley recommended forceps for speeding up labour if the woman became exhausted or distressed once the baby's head lay low in the pelvis. With judicious use, he believed that trauma to both parties was no greater than with a natural delivery. The Wrigley's fitted the bill in the 1930s when practically every general practitioner delivered babies. You couldn't apply these forceps too high, you had to pull just below where the shanks crossed, and you couldn't pull excessively. Perhaps most important of all, the fetal head couldn't be compressed too tightly.

In hindsight, perhaps it was at one time a little too easy to use Wrigley's. Armed with them, a doctor could elbow the midwife aside at the last minute to lift the baby out. It was also whispered that obstetricians in the US sometimes deployed them as a method of boosting their fees. Wrigley himself did not much profit from his invention. Despite the many thousands produced, he received no royalties.

His forceps endure today and are most often used during caesarean section if manual delivery of the head is a challenge. That was not Wrigley's only contribution to his speciality. He was a key contributor to the first four reports of the Confidential Enquiry into Maternal Deaths in England and Wales between 1953 and 1965, a national programme that is just as valuable these days as it was when it began. In his spare time, he was a fisherman and a model train buff. Wrigley was a down-to-earth Northerner who preferred using his own head and his hands. He retired in his early sixties, disenchanted with increasing technology in obstetrics.

By then, childbirth was well and truly medicalized – and masculinized. What was once an all-female province had fallen to the patriarchy. By 1886, the Medical Acts Amendment Act obliged all doctors to be examined in midwifery. And they needed to. It was an essential skill for general practitioners, who were heavily involved in labour. Before the advent of the National Health Service in 1948, it was also a reliable source of income for GPs.

❦

Obstetric forceps have always been controversial. When is it wise to leave things to nature, and when it is better to intervene? The death of twenty-one-year-old Princess Charlotte in 1817 illustrates the dilemma. Some two weeks after her due date, Princess Charlotte, George IV's only child, was in labour with her first baby. In attendance was Sir Richard Croft (1762–1818), an eminent *accoucheur* who was the great Thomas Denman's protégé as well as his son-in-law. The first stage of the princess's labour lasted twenty-six hours. Croft diagnosed that the baby was lying transversely, and sent for physician and man-midwife John Sims (1749–1831). When Sims arrived seven hours later, the princess was still labouring, but it seems that instruments to speed up her labour hadn't been considered. After seventeen more hours, a stillborn baby boy was delivered, weighing nine pounds, which seems far heavier than was predicted. Princess Charlotte herself died six hours later. This left King George without an heir, so the crown went to his brother, and then to his niece, better known in the history books as Queen Victoria. As for Croft, he was widely criticized, even though forceps may not have saved the princess. When he faced a similar situation three months later, he killed himself.

Even today, it's impossible to give a figure as to what proportion of vaginal births 'ought to be' instrumental. In the recent past, forceps have sometimes been used a little too enthusiastically. In the interests of saving precious time, for instance, a rushed mid-twentieth-century doctor might have resorted to forceps instead of waiting any longer for the baby's head to emerge.

This was massive medicalization of a normal biological process. In the twentieth century, there was even a vogue for prophylactic forceps delivery, also known as *accouchement forcé* or forcible delivery. It became popular among American obstetricians, although the concept itself went back to French barber-surgeon Ambroise Paré in the sixteenth century (see Chapter 2, page 33). *Accouchement forcé* could include forcible dilatation of the cervix, cervical incisions, routine episiotomy, and forceps. Drugs like oxytocin and prostaglandins were used to expedite delivery. There was no attempt to use posture or other natural methods of assisting the woman's efforts, like allowing her to walk about. It was the doctors who were active in labour.

At first, *accouchement forcé* was only for complex cases, but its use spread. It usually went hand in hand with pain relief in the form of so-called twilight sleep with morphine and scopolamine. It was pain relief in name only. This drug combination caused amnesia rather than anaesthesia. Under the influence of twilight sleep, women often screamed in agony. Some became delirious or violent. If they thrashed about or banged their heads, staff would restrain them. The next day, or maybe later, whenever the effects wore off, the mother might be surprised to find she had somehow produced a baby.

Despite the drawbacks, many women clamoured for twilight sleep. It was not enough to have a safe labour and to produce a healthy baby. Modern women wanted to be free of the horrors of the process, and their demands helped bring it into fashion. Magazine articles reported it in glowing terms, as did those who'd had twilight sleep in Germany where it was very popular with those that could afford it. Twilight sleep reduced the woman's autonomy during labour, so it's surprising that many early feminists welcomed it. Then again, some doctors strongly opposed it, which may have increased its appeal. For women, pain-free childbirth also offered the hope of feeling well enough to enjoy their newborn baby's first moments. But it didn't always happen that way. Recovery from the drugs could be slow, the woman was usually sore from a generous episiotomy, and she might have to wait several days to meet her baby while they rested their little head in the nursery.

Babies were often worse off from twilight sleep too. Both morphine and scopolamine cross the placenta and can depress the central nervous system. A baby might be drowsy and breathe irregularly. It's likely that the practice of holding a newborn upside down to slap it across the buttocks originated from this era. Despite the drawbacks, however, the use of *accouchement forcé* and twilight sleep persisted well into the mid-twentieth century. My own mother had twilight sleep for my birth.

The long-term effects of twilight sleep are worth noting too. It cemented the use of drugs in labour and, because it could only be used in hospital, it meant a move away from home births. With the woman fully recumbent and the midwife demoted further, the doctor reigned supreme in the delivery suite and had near total control over the birthing process. And what helped it happen? One can thank overly glowing media accounts of twilight sleep, and the power of public opinion.

~~⚬~~

The early to mid-twentieth century saw great enthusiasm for forceps, which were used in nearly half of all births. Midwives were less enamoured. Eventually a backlash took place against forceps, and natural childbirth came into vogue. GP Grantly Dick Read (1890–1959) wrote two groundbreaking books on the subject. *Natural Childbirth* in 1933 and then *Childbirth without Fear* in 1942 both helped his ideas gain traction. He advocated a gentle labour with a relaxed mother, alert enough to enjoy wondrous first moments with her baby in her arms. It was no longer enough for both participants to survive. Women had to savour the experience of birth and give the baby the best start. With Dick Read, anaesthesia was not part of the plan. A woman had to conquer the pain herself.

Many feminists of the time praised Dick Read. Unlike other obstetricians, he placed the woman at the centre of childbirth. He also recognized the vicious cycle of fear-tension-pain. Nonetheless, he was a chauvinist who was known to blame women for imagining labour pain. In his view, 'primitive women', whatever that meant, suffered no pain in childbirth. As a devout Catholic, Dick Read also caused ripples when he left his wife and children in the UK in favour of marrying his nurse and moving to South Africa.

In the 1970s, radical feminism made its mark. This movement maintained that there was systematic oppression of women throughout all cultures, and that it had existed for all time. The oppression was based on the completely wrong-headed notion of male superiority (which inevitably also meant medical superiority). Accounts of childbirth from a feminist point of view had been all too rare. Now they grew in number. Why have an instrumental delivery? After all, it was, according to many, yet one more manifestation of the patriarchy. Even female body parts were all named after men, such as the pouch of Douglas (James Douglas, 1675–1742), Fallopian tubes (Gabriele Falloppio, 1522–62), Graafian follicles in the ovary (Reinier de Graaf, 1641–73), and Bartholin's glands (Caspar Bartholin the Younger, 1655–1738).

Our Bodies, Ourselves was one of the most influential books of 1970 and has been through many editions since. Still available today, this feminist classic was first published by a non-profit organization, the Boston Women's Health Book Collective. It covers sexual health, birth control, pregnancy, abortion, childbirth, abuse, and the menopause, among other topics, and emphasizes a woman's authority

and experience in all these matters. While it places reproduction at the heart of a woman's sphere, the book's focus is
very much opposed to society's traditional view that women
should be meek and submissive. Via *Our Bodies, Ourselves*,
and in other works, conferences, and consciousness-
raising activities, women found a voice and they used it to
express their opinions on the management of labour.

Forceps can have adverse effects for both mother and baby.
Whether or not they call themselves feminists, women
often dislike the prospect of a forceps delivery. Opinions
differ according to culture and customs, as well as with
ethnicity and educational status. A US study from 2021
suggests that white women with a college education and
private health insurance view forceps more kindly, but
overall most women had a negative opinion.

Today, forceps use has dwindled and comprises a lower
proportion of vaginal deliveries. For one thing, it became
clear that there was a climate of unnecessary intervention.
For another, there are now other options. Swedish professor
Tage Malmström (1911–95) came up with the ventouse in
the 1950s as the modern version of the vacuum extractor.
Many since Simpson had worked on vacuum devices, with
Malmström's being the most successful. His model had a
cup with a rounded incurved margin to reduce the risk of it
detaching during traction.

The ventouse and forceps aren't interchangeable. While
the ventouse causes less trauma than forceps to the woman,
it is less consistent at achieving delivery. It was slow to gain

ground in Britain, but eventually became more popular in the late twentieth century. Like any instrument, it has its drawbacks, especially for the baby, such as jaundice and a lump called a chignon on the baby's head. This usually subsides within two days. The most important thing to know is that the ventouse is unsuitable for babies under thirty-five weeks' gestation because they have a greater risk of brain haemorrhage.

There is also caesarean section (C-section). Although it was occasionally used in classical times, Julius Caesar was not born this way. The word caesarean apparently comes from the Latin verb *caedere,* meaning to cut. For some centuries, the function of a caesarean was probably not to save the woman's life, let alone the child's. It was to comply with religious decrees that mother and baby be buried separately.

The first successful caesarean is often attributed to a Swiss swineherd by the name of Jakob Nufer (dates unknown). Nufer had a little knowledge of anatomy and was used to castrating pigs, so he put his instruments to work in 1500, when, it is said, his wife, Elisabeth, had laboured for several days and already seen thirteen midwives. Nufer operated and delivered a baby who went on to live into his seventies. Nufer's wife allegedly had five successful vaginal deliveries afterwards, including twins, all of which sounds a little unlikely.

In Ireland, Mary Donally almost certainly carried out the first caesarean in which the woman survived. Again, this was without anaesthetic. Donally (dates unknown) was an illiterate but experienced midwife. In 1738, she was faced with farmer's wife Alice O'Neill, aged thirty-three, who had been in labour for twelve days. The baby had perished by then, but Donally felt she had to do something. So she performed a caesarean on the woman, suturing the uterus and skin as best she could, and finally dressing the wound with egg white. O'Neill recovered within a few weeks. She did, however, have a large abdominal hernia that restricted her mobility. A firm and generous bandage was applied to hold in her intestines. As ever, the overriding principle was to get a woman back on her feet to look after the household and the other children.

For some time, a C-section was highly risky. In 1884, a review of over 100 cases revealed a maternal mortality of more than 50 per cent. With anaesthesia, antisepsis, and antibiotics when needed, the procedure is obviously far safer nowadays. While a caesarean is not interchangeable with a forceps delivery, there are some situations where operating can avoid an instrumental vaginal birth. It can also be deployed in advance of labour if problems are predictable. As caesareans became more common, and the ventouse gained ground, obstetricians in training soon had fewer opportunities to learn to use forceps safely.

Is it worth trying to keep up the forceps skills of practising doctors or should this mode of delivery be left to the past? In the current medico-legal climate, obstetrics seems to be heading in a forceps-free direction, and caesarean birth is ever more common. But if obstetricians no longer retain forceps skills, women will suffer.

The right answer isn't clear, and opinions are often polarized. That's no surprise. Birth is an emotive topic. Since the beginning of humanity, reproduction has embodied a woman's essence. Pregnancy is not a disease, as we all know. It's a natural condition. Yet women and their babies can still die during or just after the birth.

The fact is that a woman's pelvis is barely wide enough for a full-term baby's head. Human infants have correspondingly larger brains and skulls than other mammals, and, thanks to being upright, human females have a smaller pelvis. That's why, to be born at all, babies need to leave the womb at a less mature stage than, say, foals or lambs. Even so, human birth is a tight fit. That journey down the birth canal is the most treacherous voyage a person will ever make. The bottom line is that a normal birth can only be diagnosed in retrospect. While it's possible to deliver safely at home, one cannot predict how things will turn out.

For many, birth has become more high-tech than ever, with continuous fetal monitoring during labour and even intra-partum ultrasound scans. What is the optimal way to give birth? That's still an open question. Medical staff should recognize and respect female autonomy while ensuring safety for mother and baby, but sometimes those two aims don't match.

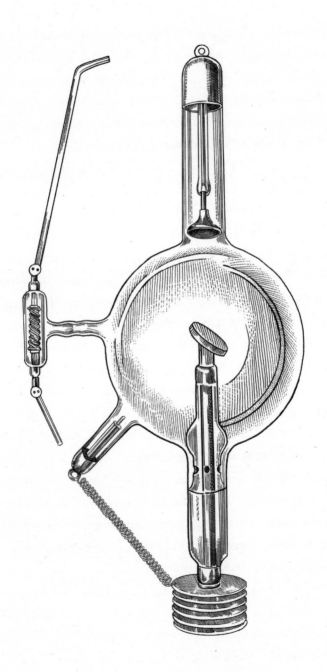

9

The X-Ray Machine: Making the Body Transparent

Medical imaging has brought benefits to millions by making use of the awesome fundamental particles in our world. This speciality is an imaginative blend of physics and biology. I think it is one of the most exciting areas of medical history.

It all began with X-rays. As with so many great discoveries, this one was accidental. On 8 November 1895, German physicist Wilhelm Conrad Roentgen (1845– 1923) was investigating cathode rays in his lab, using a Crookes tube. A Crookes tube is a glass tube containing two electrodes, positive and negative, in a partial vacuum. When a high voltage is applied between the electrodes, the remaining gases in the tube glow, thanks to a rapid beam of electrons, also known as cathode rays. Roentgen had worked hard to get this far. As a teenager, he had been expelled from school for drawing a caricature of one of the teachers. It was another student's handiwork, but Roentgen refused to tell on him. After that, it was a struggle to get into university to study engineering, and then to gain his PhD and become professor of physics at the Julius Maximilians University of Würzburg.

Cathode rays had not long been discovered and were a hot area for study at the time. Roentgen wondered whether the rays could pass through the glass of their Crookes tube. He covered the tube with black cardboard, but a nearby fluorescent screen glowed all the same. Something was escaping through the cardboard. The details of the discovery are a little sketchy because Roentgen ordered his lab notes to be burnt when he died, but his biographers agree that's what happened.

Roentgen barely left his lab for the next six weeks. He missed meals and slept on a cot by the lab bench as he tried to work out what the rays could go through, other than cardboard. He tried a book, some wood, rubber, a deck of cards, and various metal sheets. Only lead stopped the rays completely. When his wife visited the lab, by now curious to find out what had been keeping him so busy, he asked her to hold out a photographic plate in front of the beam. This produced an image of her hand, complete with the bones of her fingers and the ring she was wearing. The iconic X-ray made Roentgen's name go down in history.

He didn't know what the rays were, so he called them 'X'. Roentgen published his discovery that same year, and it made the headlines. Public speculation went wild. Could peeping toms use the rays for peering through women's knickers? In response to this fear, one London manufacturer began making lead-lined underwear.

With Crookes tubes in common use, others repeated Roentgen's experiment and the new X-rays were exploited in double-quick time. Doctors soon saw the benefits of making the body transparent. The first clinical X-ray was in January 1896 in Birmingham, when a doctor called John Hall-Edwards (1858–1926) took an image of a sterile needle stuck in the hand of his assistant. Hall-Edwards already had an interest in photography. He went on to take many more radiographs during his career, and he also became the first to use X-rays during surgery.

In the US, the first medical X-ray was in February 1896. The patient was a boy with an injured wrist. Luckily, the doctor had a brother who was an astronomer and able to oblige with an X-ray photo. It clearly showed the boy's fractured forearm.

During the Spanish-American War in 1898, attempts were made to X-ray injured soldiers to search for embedded bullets, but the exposure time needed was thirty minutes. By then, the casualty might have succumbed. Still, the possibilities of the new technology seemed endless, and it was deployed without much caution. X-rays weren't just used for diagnosis. They were also used to treat a miscellany of conditions. Doctors used them to burn off moles and relieve skin conditions ranging from acne to TB of the skin.

Roentgen found that prolonged X-ray exposure caused dermatitis, burns, ulceration, and hair loss. Hall-Edwards had to have his left arm amputated below the elbow when he developed cancer. He then lost four fingers from his right hand, leaving him with just one thumb. His left hand is kept in the Chamberlain Museum of Pathology at the University of Birmingham.

Roentgen received the first Nobel Prize for Physics in 1901. In his honour, the roentgen is a unit of radiation exposure, while roentgenology is a cumbersome US term for radiology. First created in 1994, the synthetic element roentgenium (Rg, with atomic number 111) is also named after him. It is highly radioactive and can only be created in a lab. The most stable of its known isotopes has a half-life of just two minutes.

More was to come. French physicist and engineer Antoine Henri Becquerel (1852–1908) made a major finding only weeks after Roentgen's discovery. Becquerel came from an affluent family that included generations of prominent physicists. His particular distinction was to be the first person to discover radioactivity, or at least according to most versions of history.

In 1896, Becquerel was investigating the properties of uranium salts. He believed that they could absorb radiation and then emit it as X-rays. But, when he repeated his experiment on a cloudy day, he found that his uranium gave off radiation without receiving any external stimulation. Becquerel studied this further and got the credit for discovering radioactivity. But he wasn't the first. Abel Niépce de Saint-Victor (1805–70) was a French photographer and inventor with a lab near Paris. In 1857, when he was busy working on colour photography, he found that uranium salts could expose photographic emulsions.

Although he published his findings, history has some-how forgotten him. There are, however, suggestions that Becquerel may have known of his work.

Once Becquerel published his own findings, his impetus dwindled. But all was not lost because his discovery encouraged others. In 1897 Marie Curie (1867–1934) chose uranium as the topic for her doctoral thesis. In 1898, German chemist Gerhard Carl Schmidt (1865–1949) found a second element, thorium, to be radioactive. More elements followed in quick succession.

When Becquerel died of a heart attack at the age of fifty-five, he had severe burns, not just from handling radioactive materials like radium, but from often forgetting them in his pocket. The SI unit for radioactivity, the becquerel (Bq), is named after him, and so is the uranium-rich mineral becquerelite. There are boulevards to his name in many French towns. In the heavens, minor planet 6914 is called Becquerel, and there is a Becquerel crater on the Moon and another one on Mars. Alas for Abel Niépce de Saint-Victor, nothing much seems to be named after him.

❧

Husband and wife Pierre and Marie Curie made one of the most remarkable research teams ever. Born Maria Salomea Skłodowska, Marie Curie became the first woman to win a Nobel Prize, the first person to win twice, and the only person to win a Nobel Prize in two scientific areas, physics and chemistry. As a woman, she was forbidden to go to university in her native Poland, so she went to study Paris in 1891. It was an exhilarating experience that set her on her life's work. In 1895 she married physicist Pierre Curie (1859–1906). They spent most of their marriage in the lab, researching side by side.

Marie Curie's first major discovery came when she noticed that the mineral ore pitchblende, containing uranium, was four times as active as uranium itself. That led her to suspect it might also contain another radioactive element, as yet unknown. The Curies worked on isolating it. In 1898, they announced the discovery of polonium, named after Marie's mother country. But there was more to come. The leftover pitchblende was still extremely radioactive. After a few more months' work, they found small amounts of yet another element, many times more radioactive than uranium. The Curies had found radium. The amounts of radium they isolated were tiny, but even so they both burned themselves accidentally by carrying vials of it in their pockets. Their discoveries also demonstrated something fundamental about matter; they showed that something was going on within the atom. Atoms were not indivisible after all.

In 1903, the Nobel Prize for Physics went to Pierre Curie, Henri Becquerel, and Marie Curie for their research into radiation phenomena. French scientists had originally put forward only the first two names, but protests from Pierre Curie and others ensured that Marie Curie also shared the award.

Pierre's work soon came to an end. In 1906, he was knocked down and killed by a horse and cart. Marie was

THE X-RAY MACHINE

offered his chair, becoming the first female professor at
Sorbonne University. Her work continued apace. It was
she who coined the term radioactivity. In 1911 Marie
Curie received her second Nobel Prize, this time in chemistry, for her work in measuring radioactivity. That same
year, the Sorbonne and the Pasteur Institute helped fund
her Radium Institute.

Curie was more than a brilliant researcher. As director
of the Red Cross Radiology Service during the First World
War, she developed mobile X-ray units, known as *petites
Curies*, that could be deployed to the front. Along with
her elder daughter, Irène, she set off. They both worked at
casualty triage stations, X-raying the wounded for fractures and shrapnel. Irène taught herself how to repair the
equipment, and taught doctors how best to use radiology.

These key discoveries at the end of the nineteenth century
changed both diagnosis and treatment. Marie Curie was
quick to see potential uses for radium, which soon became
a useful external treatment for cancer. As early as 1899,
two Swedish general practitioners became the first doctors
on record to use X-rays for skin tumours on the face, in
fifty separate treatment sessions for one patient and ninety-
nine for the other. There were few ways to measure the
dose, and not much in the way of safety precautions.

The treatment could be in the form of external beam
radiation or as brachytherapy (*brachy* being Greek for
'near' or 'short'). In the early days of radiotherapy, the
active agent was often applied directly to the surface of

the tumour or else within the body cavity, such as the womb. From the 1910s, doctors also began instilling the radioactive agents deep into the cancer itself. Tumours of the breast, prostate, and brain were most often treated this way.

Radiotherapy was also used indiscriminately for conditions such as epilepsy, acne, and varicose veins, even though harmful effects were becoming impossible to ignore. One man decided to investigate, on himself, the impact of radioactivity on his head. He lost all his hair in the process. More serious dangers emerged over time at even greater cost to patients, doctors, and radiographers. Benign menstrual bleeding was still being treated with radiation in the 1940s. Unfortunately, it sometimes led to cervical cancer.

In fluoroscopy, a continuous X-ray image appears on a screen. The method has many applications and has been especially useful for patients with TB. However, if they were treated with artificial lung collapse (pneumothorax), as was common in the early twentieth century, they might have frequent fluoroscopy exams, each of which delivers more radiation than a regular chest X-ray. Research has now shown a higher incidence of breast cancer in women who went through this routine.

The Second World War and the bombing of Hiroshima and Nagasaki increased concerns about radiation exposure. Even so, fluoroscopy machines were still used nonchalantly in shoe shops as an aid to fitting, especially for children whose feet grew rapidly. Concerns appeared in the *British Medical Journal* in 1950 but the machines were not banned until well after that.

～∞～

Could there be a way of imaging without the hazards of radiation? Here is where ultrasound comes in, a technique that uses waves of a frequency well above the range of hearing. Today, ultrasound is so widely used it's easy to forget how new this method is, and how quickly it became accepted despite the doubters and dissenters.

Medical ultrasound scanning was first developed by British physician Ian Donald (1910–87). At the beginning of the Second World War, Donald served as a medical officer in the RAF, where he gained experience with radar and sonar. Afterwards, as a professor of midwifery in Glasgow, he became intrigued by the possibilities of ultrasound, especially after a patient introduced him to her husband. The man was a director of the engineering company Babcock & Wilcox, which used ultrasound to check welding for flaws. Donald wanted to see whether the same technique might differentiate between various human tissues. In July 1955, Donald and a colleague arrived at the factory with their cars loaded with samples from patients, including uterine fibroids and a large cyst of the ovary. Thanks to an obliging Babcock employee, Donald got ultrasound images of his samples and his own thumb, and, as a bonus, a huge steak that the company had kindly supplied for comparison.

Could this industry-based method work on living patients? The idea was simple enough, but it required a lot

of work to put it into practice. One of the most convinc-
ing demonstrations of ultrasound came when Donald used
his machine on a sixty-four-year-old woman who was
believed to be dying of stomach cancer. Her own doctor
had already made the diagnosis with a barium X-ray
in which she drank a barium solution to delineate the
stomach on X-ray. Donald applied the ultrasound probe.
Donald's assistant, the obstetrician John MacVicar (1927–
2011), remarked that the image looked like a cyst. Donald
apologized to colleagues for his friend's outlandish suggestion. However, when Donald operated on the patient, he
found that MacVicar had been right. It was a huge benign
cyst. The patient survived and, as MacVicar said at a
symposium years later, she also sent Donald a cake every
Christmas after that.

Ultrasound images improved vastly once the so-called
B-scanner was developed, with its two-dimensional
pictures. The new device was first tested on MacVicar's
abdomen. Most of the scans thereafter were on pregnant women, the main focus of the team's work. Soon,
ultrasound was used to estimate the due date, localize
the placenta, diagnose pregnancy loss, detect twin pregnancy, and monitor fetal growth and development. When
it came into standard clinical use in the 1970s, the technique transformed antenatal care. Best of all, ultrasound
used no radiation. What about safety? It is impossible
to prove a negative, but animal experiments and long
clinical use of ultrasound since then suggest that it causes
no harm.

Ultrasound has gone on to prove its diagnostic worth beyond obstetrics. It has diagnostic uses in soft tissue conditions, biliary disease, and cardiac disorders, to mention a few examples. But there remained a need for something more.

⌖

The simplest description of computerized axial tomography (known as CT or CAT scanning) is that it is an offshoot of regular X-rays, but it's a touch more complex than that. CT scans came into being in the 1960s thanks to British electrical engineer Godfrey Hounsfield (1919–2004). The youngest of five children of a farming family, Hounsfield grew up in a rural childhood idyll. He had no great academic inclination but he loved being out of doors. There was also the lure of the machinery on the farm. Before his teens, he was experimenting with his own contraptions. In his autobiography, he recalls making his own recording devices, throwing himself off haystacks with an improvised glider, and almost killing himself when he used water-filled tar barrels and acetylene to see how high they could be waterjet propelled.

In the RAF, Hounsfield learned about electronics and radar. After the Second World War, he gained a diploma in electrical engineering, then began work at EMI in London. There were two strands to EMI's work, electronics and music – hence 'Electrical and Musical Industries'. Hounsfield's interest was computing. In 1958, he helped devise the first commercially available all-transistor British computer, the EMIDEC 1100. Come 1967, EMI gave Hounsfield carte blanche to develop a product of his own choice. We may have The Beatles to thank for the CT scanner. The spectacular success of the Fab Four's music had filled EMI's coffers, which enabled the company to allow Hounsfield such freedom.

On a long country ramble, Hounsfield came up with an idea. He reckoned one could figure out what was inside a closed box by taking X-rays at various angles through it. He went on to build a computer that could receive input from a multitude of X-rays and then put together a 3D image of the object in a series of cross-sections. This is the essence of computerized tomography.

Hounsfield built a prototype scanner and tested it first on a preserved human brain, then on fresh animal parts. He travelled across London by public transport with carrier bags of his specimens, including a cow brain from a Kosher slaughterhouse in East London, and various parts of pig bodies. For the first live human scan, Hounsfield used his own head.

Those early images needed a scanning time of many hours, which was not workable for patients. But Hounsfield managed to shorten it to just over four minutes. In 1971 at the Atkinson Morley Hospital in South London, a forty-one-year-old woman with a suspected brain tumour became the first patient to have the scan. The image revealed a suspicious lesion. The surgeon who then operated said his findings looked exactly like the scan.

Next came a whole-body scanner in 1975. The images were remarkably clear, with shading in the pictures representing tissue density. With further refinements, the computer even produced colour images. Meanwhile, South African Allan Cormack had been working on the theoretical maths for CT scanning. Allan MacLeod Cormack (1924–98) was mainly a nuclear physicist with an interest in tomography. His work proved integral to the scanner. In 1979, Hounsfield and Cormack jointly received the Nobel Prize in Physiology or Medicine.

EMI scanning, as it was first called, has since been used on most parts of the body. Its pictures are precise and its uses are legion. Since it gives off X-rays, however, it is not always the best method for repeat imaging, or for screening in the absence of symptoms.

Hounsfield's name is immortalized in the Hounsfield (symbol HU), a unit of radiodensity used for evaluating CT scans. Tales of his eccentricities live on, too. Wherever he was in the world, he insisted on keeping to the time back home. As a result, he sometimes delivered lectures at 10 a.m. Greenwich Mean Time, even if it was midnight for his audience.

The principles of computerized tomography that Hounsfield established are still in use today. But his research also contributed to other imaging methods, like magnetic resonance and positron emission tomography.

❧

Instead of X-rays, positron emission tomography (PET) relies on radioactive emissions from a tracer compound. The aim is to display the activity of the brain or other organs. In other words, the technique focuses on function rather than structure. Patients receive an injection of a radioactive tracer, which different brain areas metabolize to varying extents, depending on their level of activity at the time. The radiotracer gives off positrons (positive anti-particles of electrons) that collide with electrons to produce two high energy photons, emitted at 180 degrees. Scanners arranged in a circle around the body use these photons to assess density and create an image of the blood flow and activity of that area.

Developed in the 1960s, this high-tech method required a cast of scientists worthy of a Hollywood blockbuster, plus a menagerie of animals. But the first insights that made PET scanning possible came long before the discovery of positrons in the twentieth century. In 1878, Italian phys-iologist Angelo Mosso (1846–1910) measured an increase in brain pulsations from the right prefrontal cortex during an arithmetic task by a subject with a defect of his skull bones. Fifty years later, another patient with a striking condition helped demonstrate the link between blood flow and brain function. In 1928, American neurophysiolo-gist John Farquhar Fulton (1899–1960, see Chapter 10) reported the case of a man with a vascular malformation in his occipital lobe. This produced an abnormal sound called a 'bruit'. When the patient used his eyes, the bruit became louder. Fulton became well known for localiz-ing cerebral function in primates. His work cemented the blood flow–function relationship.

The next part of the PET story concerns isotopes (or, as purists might prefer to say, radionuclides). Significant advances took place in the early twentieth century, thanks to New Zealand physicist Ernest Rutherford (1871–1937). He was the first person to set off an artificial nuclear reaction, so he is often described as the Father of Nuclear Physics. Chemist George de Hevesy (1885–1966) went to work under Rutherford at the University of Manchester. De Hevesy came from a noble Hungarian family and was miserable in Manchester. For one thing, Rutherford was setting him impossible assignments. For another, the boarding house he lived in (recommended by Rutherford himself) served unpalatable food that gave him indigestion. De Hevesy was sure leftovers were being recycled. He suggested to the landlady that she provide freshly prepared meat more than once a week. Bristling, she denied using anything other than fresh items for every meal. One Sunday in 1911, de Hevesy surreptitiously dropped a little radioactive lead onto the leftovers on his plate. Lo and behold, the detector he smuggled into the dining room a few days later showed radioactivity in the soufflé. De Hevesy had made his point.

By the 1930s, plenty more radioisotopes were on the way. Irène Joliot-Curie (1897–1956, daughter of Pierre and Marie) and her husband Frédéric (1900–58) created several more. This led to their Nobel Prize in Chemistry in 1935, making them the second married couple to be Nobel laureates. Their work launched the field of nuclear medicine.

In 1961, Danish physician Niels A. Lassen (1926–97) and Swedish physician David H. Ingvar (1924–2000) worked with radioactive krypton-85 and xenon-133 to localize sensory, motor, and cognitive functions in humans. They produced colour-coded representations of blood flow in its relation to brain function. This is still the look of cerebral PET scans today.

American physician and neuroscientist Louis Sokoloff (1921–2015) continued the work on tracers. In the mid-1940s, Sokoloff was also an army psychotherapist and chief of neuropsychiatry at Camp Lee, Virginia. He fervently believed that mental illness had physiological and biochemical components. 'Of course, the psychoanalysts said it had nothing to do with the brain,' he once said in an interview. 'It had to do with the mind – it could have been anywhere. It could have been in the big toe.'

Sokoloff's work showed that it was not in the big toe. He researched enzymes and physiology to assess brain metabolism. With radioactive 2-deoxyglucose as tracer, he made real-time images of living animal brains, revealing which areas were most active at any given time. This was the beginning of accurately mapping a live brain. Soon, it was adapted to PET scanning.

In 1976, Sokoloff was joined by radiochemists Alfred Wolf and Joanna Fowler. Together, the trio synthesized the most useful tracer of all. Alfred Peter Wolf (1923–98), usually called Al, had served in the army during the Second World War and spent time in Los Alamos on the Manhattan Project to produce the world's first nuclear weapons. After the war, he went into research. By then, he was the epitome of the cultured New Yorker, a connoisseur of food, wine, and music. But he also had a flair for chemistry. Wolf developed radiolabelling techniques by using atoms with very high energies. In this way, he created organic radiotracers, in particular 2-fluoro-2-deoxy-D-glucose (FDG). Glucose use is greatest when cells divide rapidly, as they do in cancers. Even more useful in terms of imaging, the most aggressive cancers show the highest rates of glucose metabolism. Today, FDG is still the most sensitive tracer for imaging and assessing tumours, and also helps oncologists evaluate the response to treatment.

Wolf did his work on radiotracers at Brookhaven, the lab established in Long Island after the war to explore the peaceful applications of atomic physics. He and his entourage at Brookhaven came to be known as the Wolf Pack, and scientists flocked from around the world to learn from him.

Joanna Fowler (b. 1942) was a psychiatry professor as well as director of one of Brookhaven's programmes. With radiotracers, she studied the effects of disease, drugs, and ageing on the brain. She found that smokers have reduced levels of monoamine oxidase (MAO), this being one of the chemicals that regulates neurotransmitters in the brain and other organs. Fowler's work raised interest in the link between depression and addiction to tobacco and other substances, and has led to further research.

Prototype PET scanners were developed in the early 1960s, and further research enabled more advances in both radiotracers and instruments. It's impossible to go through the entire roll call of distinguished scientists who helped develop PET. However, I cannot leave out award-winning

US physicist Michael E. Phelps (b. 1939). One of eight children, Phelps had it tough. His father was disabled with a broken back. When Phelps was nine, a fire destroyed their home, killing two of his brothers and severely burning his mother. As a young adult, Phelps took up boxing, initially to help channel his anger. But at nineteen, a car crash put him in a coma for days. It was the loss of his future as a boxer, but it was science's gain. Phelps went to Western Washington University where he got his degree in chemistry and maths.

He worked on positron decay as well as a detection system and the electronics needed to build a 3D image. By 1973, Phelps put all this together into the first PET scanner. The first whole-body PET scanner appeared in 1977. But research wasn't his whole life. Phelps founded and then directed the first PET clinic aimed exclusively at patient care. It focused on diagnosing conditions such as Alzheimer's disease, multi-infarct dementia, Parkinson's disease, the inherited disorder Huntington's disease, epilepsy, depression, heart disease, and cancers. No wonder he is the person most often named as the inventor of PET.

⤝⤞

PET is not the only imaging technique that uses radioactive compounds. In 1950, Benedict Cassen (1902–72), a physicist at the University of California, developed the first radioisotope imaging system. His scintiscanner combined a Geiger counter with crystal components of a photomultiplier tube to detect gamma ray emissions. After giving a person radioiodine, which has an affinity for the thyroid gland, Cassen's scanner could image the gland to spot suspicious lumps and the like. Exactly the same principle applies to scanning other parts of the body, using radioactive compounds aimed at that specific organ. This elegant technique proved incredibly useful from the early 1950s until the mid-1970s, when CT scanning arrived on the scene.

It gets even more complicated when you consider single photon emission computed tomography (SPECT). PET uses positrons, as its name suggests, while SPECT measures gamma rays from radioactive tracer molecules administered to the patient. SPECT scanning helps diagnose and follow up heart diseases, such as blocked coronary arteries. With different radiotracers, it can also be applied to bone disease, gall bladder disorders, and bleeding from the gut. More recently, SPECT has become valuable in Parkinson's disease and dementia, as well as for various cancers.

If PET and SPECT are hard to grasp, get ready for magnetic resonance imagining (MRI). Unlike CT, it does not involve X-rays. So how does MRI work?

MRI scanners create a strong magnetic field that forces protons (hydrogen ions) in the body to align in that field. Radiofrequency waves are then pulsed through the patient, which stimulates the protons out of equilibrium. When the radio waves are turned off, the protons spring back to their position and send back radio signals. As protons in different parts of the body resume their alignment in the magnetic field, sensors measure the time taken and the amount of energy released. The faster the protons realign, the brighter the image.

The differences between tissues enable the scanner to build up images. Most MRI machines are tube-shaped magnets within which the patient lies. When you're inside the machine, the magnetic field works with radio waves and hydrogen atoms in the body to create cross-sectional images, like slices in a loaf of bread. It feels just as claustrophobic as being inside a bread bin, and it's considerably noisier.

Since MRI doesn't use radiation, it's ideal when repeated imaging is needed, especially within the brain. It's better than CT for many purposes, but it costs more. There are new magnetic resonance techniques too, such as MRI angiography (MRA) to assess blood flow through arteries.

As you might expect, many people worked on the development of this sophisticated technique. In fact, the history of MRI began nearly a century ago, with Austrian-born physicist Isidor Isaac Rabi (1898–1988). Rabi was still an infant when his family moved to New York in 1899. He got a degree in chemistry but fell in love with physics. After finishing his PhD in 1927, he went to Europe and spent time working with the biggest names in quantum physics, including Niels Bohr (1885–1962), Wolfgang Pauli (1900–58), Otto Stern (1888–1969), Werner Heisenberg (1901–76), and Erwin Schrödinger (1887–1961).

The quantum bug bit. His parents were Orthodox Jews, but Rabi did not practise. Physics was his religion.

When he returned to the USA, he set up a molecular beam lab and spent time researching the nuclear spin of atoms. He found that radio waves could force magnetic atomic nuclei to flip their orientation, and then give off energy on return to their normal state. That phenomenon is nuclear magnetic resonance, for which he was awarded the 1944 Nobel Prize in Physics.

Whereas Rabi had studied molecular beams, Edward Purcell and Felix Bloch independently worked on magnetic resonance within solids and liquids. Edward Mills Purcell (1912–97) was a US physicist inspired by Rabi. He worked with nuclear magnetism at Harvard, where he was a professor. Felix Bloch (1905–83) was a Swiss-American physicist who had learned from some of the finest minds in the business, like Werner Heisenberg, Niels Bohr, and Enrico Fermi (1901–54). He left Europe when the Nazis took power in 1933. After becoming an American citizen, he worked on atomic energy at Los Alamos during the Second World War. Later, he became the first head of CERN, the European Organisation for Nuclear Research, now home to the Large Hadron Collider. In 1946, Bloch and Purcell separately developed methods to study different materials. They were awarded their Nobel Prize in Physics in 1952.

Nuclear magnetic resonance imaging (NMRI), as it was then called, was mainly a chemistry tool at first. It took a lot more work during the 1970s before it became useful for patients.

American chemist Paul Lauterbur (1929–2007) had a lifelong passion for science. As a teenager, he built a lab at home in the basement. At school, his chemistry teacher let him carry out his own experiments at the back of the class. His idea for MRI came to him one day when he was with a colleague at a Big Boy restaurant in Pittsburgh. On his second bite into their signature burger, Lauterbur had his brainwave and began scribbling on a napkin. Soon he rushed out of the restaurant to get a notebook from a nearby drugstore. He spent most of the night filling its pages with his thoughts on taking MRI pictures of the human body. Back at the State University of New York, he initially tested his theory with tubes of heavy water and plain water. When he submitted his findings to *Nature*, the journal rejected his paper. 'Anything new is likely to meet a certain amount of incomprehension at first,' he said. 'Many said it couldn't be done, even when I was doing it.'

At around the same time, British physicist Peter Mansfield (1933–2017) was also working on nuclear magnetic resonance (NMR). Unlike Lauterbur, Mansfield came late to science, thanks to a careers teacher who told him that science wasn't for him, a prediction that turned out to be somewhat wide of the mark. He left school at fifteen with no qualifications and became an apprentice printer. Then he read an article about a boy who'd worked in rocket propulsion at RAF Westcott, Buckinghamshire. He wrote to find out more, and landed a job at Westcott in 1952.

Mansfield passed his O-level exams at evening classes. He then studied for A-levels in physics and maths during his military service. With encouragement from the staff at Westcott, he studied physics at university. He got a first-class degree in 1959 and went on to do a PhD. From then on, there was no stopping him.

He devoted the rest of his career to NMR. In the early 1970s, NMR was deployed in almost every chemistry department, but nobody imagined that it could be used for anatomical imaging. For one thing, the scanners were painfully slow. But Mansfield's innovations, including a technique called echo-planar imaging (EPI), turned scanners into high-speed machines and made clinical use realistic. At the University of Nottingham in 1978, Mansfield tested the first full body prototype of what was then called NMR. Despite fearing a heart attack from the procedure, he volunteered to be the guinea pig and thereby produced the first scan of a live person. That prototype is now an exhibit in the Science Museum, London.

By the way, NMR was the original name for the new scanning technique, but it soon changed to magnetic resonance imaging (MRI), a term that avoids some of the negative undertones of the word 'nuclear'. These days, nobody seems that worried about the word. Hospital departments that deal with imaging methods such as SPECT are now often called Nuclear Medicine.

Mansfield's echo-planar imaging (EPI) technique also led to functional MRI (fMRI), in which the brain can be imaged during specific tasks to determine the precise location of a specific function, such as speech or memory. The task may be moving fingers or toes, listening to speech, or reciting a well-known rhyme. In 2003, when Mansfield was seventy, he and Lauterbur shared the Nobel prize in Physiology or Medicine for their work on MRI. The teenager once deemed unsuitable for science now has an asteroid named after him.

It was Raymond Damadian, however, who produced the first commercial MRI scanning machine. Raymond Vahan Damadian (1936–2022) was an Armenian-American physician. He was ten when his beloved grandmother died of breast cancer. He was a gifted violinist, but medical innovation became his passion from that point on.

In the late 1960s, he worked on NMR effects at the cellular level. He demonstrated that tumour cells in mice showed a longer relaxation time than normal cells. A little later, he set about building a scanner for human use. In refining the technique, he and his team turned again to hapless rodents. In 1976, they produced an image of a tumour in the chest of a mouse. Of course, they knew the tumour was there. They had implanted it.

In July 1977, one of Damadian's slimmer colleagues underwent the first human MRI body scan. It took nearly five hours to produce a very basic picture. All the same, the machine had achieved what many said was impossible. The team named the scanner 'Indomitable'. The following year, Damadian founded the FONAR Corporation to produce the scanner (FONAR being field focusing nuclear magnetic resonance). But it didn't sell, and Damadian's brainchild ended up in the Smithsonian Institution in

Washington, DC. FONAR went on to manufacture the first commercial MRI scanner in 1980, and many since then. However, it was the methods developed by Lauterbur and Mansfield that endured.

Nobel Prize rules allow for an award to be shared by up to three people, but that did not happen in 2003 when the physics prize went to Lauterbur and Mansfield. Damadian was incensed. He suggested that Lauterbur and Mansfield should have refused the prize unless he, too, was given recognition. Actually, he believed that credit should go to him, and then Lauterbur, presumably bypassing Mansfield. Meanwhile, Lauterbur thought that only *he* should get credit. Right after the Nobel announcement, a group called 'The Friends of Raymond Damadian' placed full-page advertisements in the *New York Times*, the *Washington Post*, the *Los Angeles Times*, and *Dagens Nyheter*, a leading Swedish newspaper. The headline told of 'The Shameful Wrong That Must Be Righted', but the Nobel Committee would not backtrack.

MRI has gone on to flourish. Combining PET with CT or MRI, doctors can visualize both function and anatomy, and keep radiation doses low. But imaging is not only remarkable for its stunning views of the living body. MRI, for instance, can also be used to study objects such as fossils and mummies.

More significantly, making the body see-through has launched the speciality of interventional radiology. Imaging, whether by X-ray or one of the other methods, enables procedures that were previously undreamed of. Simple examples are ultrasound-guided needle biopsy of a breast lump and chorionic villus sampling in pregnancy. There's also angioplasty, in which a balloon-tipped catheter is inflated to widen a blocked artery and to place a stent to keep it patent.

The procedure known as therapeutic embolization is the opposite. Through a catheter, a specialist inserts a glue-like fluid to stop blood flow in that vessel. This technique can control bleeding, treat a vascular malformation, or even enable the non-surgical removal of a spleen or a kidney. Imaging has also widened the repertoire in oncology. Now some treatments can be introduced directly into the cancer. Then there's ultrasound-guided surgery on the fetus for complications like twin-to-twin transfusion syndrome.

Imaging can be expensive, which limits its availability. As ever, those able to afford it are not necessarily those who need it most. At a price, anyone who wants a private MRI scan can get one, even in the absence of any symptoms. Whole-body MRI screening has been endorsed by several celebrities including Kim Kardashian, though most medics agree that they are wasteful. They can also cause anxiety if the scan picks up something that needs more tests before eventually being declared an innocent finding.

The wider use of imaging in medicine has brought immense benefits, but it has driven the focus further away from doctor–patient interaction. After all, why spend precious time asking questions or examining a patient when a high-tech scan can sort it all out? Imaging really has changed the face of medicine, and not all of it for the better.

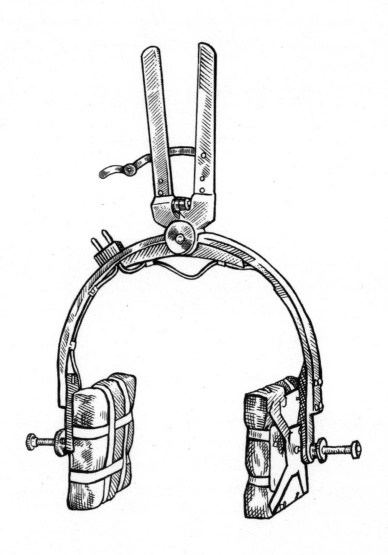

10

The ECT Machine and Shocking Approaches to Mental Illness

Psychiatry emerged as a proper specialty only in the twentieth century. Even then, it's debatable how proper it was, especially when you consider electroconvulsive treatment (ECT).

In popular depictions, a patient in a grim psychiatric ward is dragged screaming down a hallway. Once manhandled into a dingy treatment room, several people strap them down onto a gurney. Without speaking, let alone uttering a word of reassurance, the medical staff apply electrodes to either side of their head. Then, while they are still wide awake, they pass a massive jolt of electricity through their brain. The patient contorts in agony, convulses uncontrollably, and empties their bladder before passing into oblivion, quite possibly foaming at the mouth.

Fortunately, this no longer happens today. However, violent convulsions were the whole point of shock treatment. Research took off in the 1930s when Hungarian neuroscientist Ladislas (a.k.a. László) Meduna (1896–1964) searched for ways of triggering seizures in people diagnosed with schizophrenia. It seemed a promising idea at the time: since the nineteenth century, asylum staff had noticed that patients who also had epilepsy became less troublesome after having a seizure. Even more compelling, Meduna found that, at postmortem, the brains of those with epilepsy had a large number of glial cells, whereas those with schizophrenia showed the opposite. Glial cells support and maintain nerve cells, and help nerve impulses travel.

Meduna tried out various means of giving animals convulsions. After studying several chemicals, he settled on camphor mixed in oil. By 1834, he was confident enough to experiment on humans. Luck was with him and his first few patients. Nine out of those eleven happened to have a condition called catatonia. Typically, posture and movements are abnormal, and symptoms tend to improve after a seizure.

The next discovery was that high doses of pentylene-tetrazol (also called Metrazol) could trigger seizures too. And patients did sometimes improve after a convulsion induced by Metrazol. This drug was already used to stimulate breathing and the circulation, so medics already knew a lot about it. Not everything, however. Nearly half the patients convulsed so violently that they fractured their spines. Metrazol also gave them such an intense feeling of dread shortly before the seizure that they would do anything to avoid a repeat session. If doctors wanted patients to return, they had to find another way to give them convulsions.

Italian neuropsychiatrist Ugo Cerletti (1877–1963) focused on exactly this. He had studied with some of the most eminent specialists in Europe, including French neurologist Pierre Marie (1853–1940) and German psychiatrist Alois Alzheimer (1864–1915), and he had observed how nervous tissue reacts to different stimuli.

Why he decided to experiment with electric shocks isn't clear, although he came from the same proud nation that had produced the physicists Luigi Galvani (1737–98) and Alessandro Volta (1745–1827), both pioneers in electricity. According to one story, there was also a more specific reason. Cerletti allegedly wanted a particular cut of pork one day. As the butcher did not have it, they went out to the slaughterhouse where the butcher connected electrodes to the head of a live pig before he slit its throat. As he watched the violent fits, Cerletti speculated what the effect on humans might be. There's no proof that this event took place, but we do know that Cerletti embarked on experiments with electric shocks on dogs and other animals, causing repeated seizures. Many of the animals he used ended up dying. He carried on regardless for nearly a year, although he did change the positioning of the electrodes, which reduced the death rate.

In 1938, Cerletti charged his assistant Lucio Bini (1908–64) with building an apparatus to deliver therapeutic shocks to humans. As far as Cerletti was concerned, it worked like a dream. The shock put his first patient to sleep and, on waking, they had no memory of the seizure. What's more, the patient showed marked improvement.

There were precedents of sorts for the use of electricity, if one counts the electrical eels that Ancient Romans used for gout and headaches. Benjamin Franklin (1705–90) also used electricity as a treatment when he applied it to a woman with hysterical fits in the 1750s. To the shame of many nations, electric shocks were also used during the First World War for malingerers. The shocks were meant to hurt enough to convince soldiers to return to the front. However, in all of these examples it was the electrical impulse that was believed to be curative, not its convulsant effect.

If causing seizures sounds barbaric, just compare it with what came shortly beforehand. In 1927, Austrian psychiatrist Manfred Sakel (1900–57) was experimenting with the newly isolated hormone insulin when he accidently gave an overdose. His patient promptly went into a coma, but on waking he felt a lot better. This prompted Sakel to devise insulin coma therapy for schizophrenia. Patients were injected with a huge dose of insulin to induce a coma from which they would have to be rescued an hour or more later with glucose. The treatment seemed to work for some, and almost every large psychiatric hospital adopted it. It was, however, time-consuming and required close supervision. It also carried the risk of permanent neurological damage or death.

In contrast, Cerletti and Bini's *apparecchio per l'elettroshock* was a simple device with a control panel and two electrodes housed in a large headset. The panel had a power switch, a voltmeter to measure the potential difference, an ammeter to adjust the current, and a clock to fine-tune its duration in fractions of a second.

The apparatus was patented and put into wide use. Several updated versions soon followed. From the 1940s, Cerletti and Bini's technique went on to be deployed all over the world. It was less dangerous than chemicals as it caused fewer broken bones. It was also cheaper. No wonder electroconvulsive therapy, or ECT as it was called by then, replaced insulin and Metrazol and became the number one form of treatment. At the time, the indications for its use included acute schizophrenia, major depression, and manic-depressive illness (which is nowadays called bipolar disorder).

Cerletti had other interests too. He wrote widely on Alzheimer's, syphilis, and other diseases. As a medical captain in the First World War, he introduced white uniforms for troops known as the Alpini to give them better camouflage in the snow. But it was ECT that assured his fame.

Another popular treatment was prefrontal leucotomy. To give a little historical context, illustrious neurologists like Paul Broca (1824–80) and Carl Wernicke (1848–1905) had already shown that some disorders could be localized to certain parts of the brain. Surely there was an anatomical location for mental illness too?

As with ECT, animal experiments came first. American neurophysiologist and historian John Farquhar

Fulton became Yale's youngest professor in 1930. He wasted no time in building a major research lab at Yale Medical School, the first in the US to experiment on chimpanzees. Chimps Lucy and Becky both underwent removal of their frontal lobes. This left them with some memory loss and other impairments. However, what impressed Fulton was the change in their attitude and behaviour. Previously the chimps had become agitated when they failed the tests they were set. After frontal lobectomy neither Lucy nor Becky seemed to have a care in the world.

Fulton presented his work at the International Neurological Congress in London in 1935. At the conference, one of the delegates was a Portuguese neurologist with the magnificent moniker António Caetano de Abreu Freire Egas Moniz (1874–1955). He was a man of many talents, having written books on sexology, been an ambassador to Spain during the First World War, represented Portugal at the Versailles Peace Conference, and served as his country's Foreign Secretary. He had also invented cerebral angiography, which earned him two nominations for a Nobel Prize. Moniz returned to Lisbon from the congress in London excited by the prospect of applying Fulton's research to humans.

Working with neurosurgeon Pedro Almeida Lima (1903–85), he developed the subtly different operation of prefrontal leucotomy. This left the frontal lobes in place, but it severed some of their connections. Moniz and Lima also devised a leucotome, a long instrument with a steel strip for cutting into white matter. They concluded from their work on patients that prefrontal leucotomy was not only simple but failsafe. In their view, it was especially useful for depression. The Nobel Committee was equally impressed. In 1949, Moniz was awarded the Nobel Prize in Physiology or Medicine for his pioneering surgery. Later, the Nobel Foundation was pressed to rescind the award, but would not do so.

Leucotomy flourished, even if the patients didn't always. In the US, psychiatrist Walter Freeman renamed the operation lobotomy and became notorious for his enthusiasm. Walter Jackson Freeman II (1895–1972) was director of the research labs at St Elizabeth's Hospital, a large and forbidding federal mental facility in Washington, DC. It had opened in 1855 as the Government Hospital for the Insane.

There had been no controlled studies of lobotomy, nor of any other psychiatric treatments. Nonetheless, Freeman was impressed by Moniz's results. He applied the procedure to the many patients who had been at St Elizabeth's for decades without any hope of improvement. Since Freeman wasn't trained in neurosurgery, he enlisted the services of neurosurgeon James Winston Watts (1904–94). In 1936, the two men carried out the first prefrontal lobotomy in the US. Their patient was a woman in her sixties who was incapacitated by what had been diagnosed as agitated depression. Soon after the anaesthetic wore off, she was calm and couldn't even recall what she had been so apprehensive about. As with chimps Lucy and Becky, things just didn't bother her any more.

The operation may have helped some, but it was hardly failsafe. In 1941, Freeman and Watts performed a lobotomy on John F. Kennedy's sister, Rosemary Kennedy (1918–2005), who was twenty-three years old at the time. Surgery did not help. After the procedure, she could no longer walk, talk, or look after herself, and she needed care for the remaining sixty-four years of her existence.

Freeman was undeterred. In 1945, he devised a way of carrying out the procedure through the eye socket. Transorbital lobotomy needed no anaesthetic and no neurosurgeon. It could be done by psychiatrists in facilities where there were no operating rooms. A sharp instrument called an orbitoclast went in under the eyelid and from there into the brain, driven by a mallet. The instrument wasn't just inspired by an ice pick. It probably was an ice pick from the Freeman family kitchen drawer, according to his son Frank. 'We had several of them,' Frank once told a journalist. 'We used to use them to punch holes in our belts when we got bigger.'

The transorbital method played an important part in making lobotomy popular. Freeman himself performed about 100 procedures a week, wearing neither gloves nor a mask. He may also have been less than diligent in sterilizing his instruments. In 1947, his colleague Watts ended their working relationship.

Freeman continued without him, travelling across the US to various mental facilities. During his forty-year career, he is said to have carried out nearly 4,000 lobotomies. The surgery was done for a miscellany of reasons, including schizophrenia, obsessive-compulsive disorder, and post-natal depression. The diagnoses of many of the psychological disorders were not always very scientific. ECT was also used for stomach ulcers and colitis.

By 1951, over 18,000 patients in the US had had a lobotomy. The vast majority of them were adult women. Many doctors believed lobotomy was no more invasive than whipping out an inflamed appendix. Unlike appendicectomy, however, Freeman's procedure carried a mortality rate of some 15 per cent. Bleeding into the brain caused many of the deaths, but in 1951 a patient in Iowa died when Freeman paused for a photo during lobotomy, and the orbitoclast inadvertently entered too far into the brain. In 1967, he was finally banned from performing surgery, although he kept his licence to practise medicine.

In Freeman's view, psychosis was the outcome of excessive self-reflection. Severing nerve fibres could literally halt the cycle of painful thoughts whirring around the brain. Nowadays, lobotomy is considered one of the gravest mistakes of modern medicine, and I can't help wishing Freeman had self-reflected a little more.

Set against treatments like insulin coma and lobotomy, ECT seemed enlightened. In any case, the only other option for many was a life spent in an institution. With asylums full of distressed patients that nobody could help, a quick fix was very appealing.

⊰⊱

Asylums go back to the fifth century CE at least, when charitable hospitals opened for the sick, the poor, the blind, the orphaned, the needy, and various pilgrims. Many asylums were monastic foundations. As time passed, some of them focused on housing the mentally ill. Among these was London's Bethlehem Hospital, often called Bedlam, which was first founded in 1247. There wasn't much treatment on offer. Immersion in cold water was an alleged cure for madness, especially in the seventeenth century. It was a test for witches too, which says a lot about the theories of madness at the time. Lunatic asylums also provided entertainment for the well-off who came to ogle and tease the residents. Eventually the word 'bedlam' became synonymous with madness and disorder.

In the mid-nineteenth century, more and more state-funded asylums were built in Europe, Canada, and the US. They were also renamed 'mental hospitals', as if the change of name would change their ethos. Most people in the Victorian era called them madhouses regardless, and the number of inmates grew, without much being done to help them other than keeping them out of the way.

One of today's best-known psychiatric hospitals is the Maudsley in South London. Founded in 1907, it owes its existence to Henry Maudsley (1835–1918). He was a conundrum of a man, a psychiatrist who detested the word 'psychiatrist', and a doctor who treated mostly women but found them distasteful (all the more so if they gave birth). He was particularly vocal when arguing against women entering the medical profession. Thanks to his private practice, Maudsley had a vast wealth and left some £30,000 to build a hospital that would be a radical departure from the asylum organization. His vision was to treat acute mental illness, combining patient care with research and professional training. That done, he spent his last years as a recluse.

⤖

Still nobody knew what caused mental illness, but the belief persisted that insanity was some kind of disease of the body rather than the spirit. This prompted doctors to look for causes within the brain and other organs. In women, it was obvious what the trouble was. Their reproductive system sapped so much energy from the rest of the body that they were prone to mental illness at various times, such as menstruation, pregnancy, childbirth, the menopause, or any time of life, really. Symptoms of madness in women could range from irregular periods to unbecoming conduct like aggression, sexual excitement, or a liking for intellectual pursuits. Society held that a woman's identity was synonymous with her domestic function and excluded other roles. Psychiatrists went along with this. They readily treated women who had no signs of mental illness, other than refusing to submit to the ways of the world and the wishes of men in particular.

Within asylums, patients were often restrained. The straitjacket dates back to the late eighteenth century. Made of cloth (or sometimes leather), it was softer than metal restraints and seen as more humane. It was considered especially appropriate for the fairer sex. Some models covered the head or had a device that kept the legs immobile. A few even tied the wearer securely to their bed, but most straitjackets enabled patients to walk about without harming themselves or others. However, a straitjacket did not allow the wearer to eat or use the toilet unaided. Putting someone into the jacket was also traumatic, and bones often broke in the process.

Coming into this treatment vacuum, ECT reigned. In its early years, it was used for nearly every kind of mental illness, but eventually it was mostly for depressive disorders, as opposed to schizophrenia, for which it was originally developed. ECT use flourished in the mid-twentieth century. That's no surprise, perhaps, since the mid-1950s saw a bulge in patient numbers in institutions, both in the UK and the US. In the US, about 300,000 people a year underwent ECT. During the 1950s, ECT was also adopted to 'treat' homosexuality, which was considered an illness at the time.

The treatments I've described so far were not the only ones. The privileged had other options. Austrian neurologist Sigmund Freud qualified as a doctor at the University of Vienna in 1881. He formulated his theory of the unconscious and expounded a model of the psyche consisting of three parts: the id, the ego, and the superego. In his view, libido was sexualized energy that permeates all mental processes, as does the death drive.

At first, he favoured hypnosis as a treatment, but the results disappointed him. By 1896, Freud had founded psychoanalysis, a method that relies on dialogue between patient and therapist, and the use of free association.

Famously, he invented 'penis envy', for which he has received considerable criticism, not least because he took it for granted that the male was superior. Women who were frigid were, in his estimation, unable to adjust to their role as a female.

This is just a simplified view of some of Freud's work. In respect of his theories, I can't help thinking that he must have had a fertile imagination and prodigious self-belief. However, he was hardly the only medical pioneer who needed no objective evidence on which to base his beliefs. Psychiatry at that time, as at most other times, consisted largely of men pontificating on matters of which nobody knew very much.

While Freud's philosophies may not have worn well, his methods made a lasting mark on modern psychiatric practice. His system of psychoanalysis led to many later variants, all of them focused on letting patients talk freely of their problems. The mid-twentieth century saw the heyday of therapy based on Freud's work, especially in the US where the '50-minute hour' with one's analyst was a regular fixture for those able to afford it. Along with Carl Jung (1875–1961) and Alfred Adler (1870–1937), Freud left a rich legacy of talking therapies at a time when people with mental illness were barely listened to.

In the late nineteenth century, there was also the 'rest cure', the brainchild of Silas Weir Mitchell (1829–1914), American neurologist, scientist, novelist, and sometime poet. His rest cure was a treatment for 'neurasthenia', a nebulous condition widely diagnosed at the time and believed to be a depletion of nerves. Symptoms could be wide ranging but the most common were fatigue and anxiety. Alongside rest, Mitchell's prescription involved a high-protein, high-fat diet. He soon earned the nickname 'Dr Diet and Dr Quiet'. The rest cure was internationally known and extensively used, especially in more affluent circles.

∞

In the 1950s, treatment for mental illness changed dramatically with the advent of drug therapy. Several advances occurred at around the same time. The major tranquillizer chlorpromazine was discovered in 1951, during a search for a drug that would kill worms. Despite a few unwanted side effects, it made all the difference to some people with schizophrenia. Other similar drugs have been developed since, including long-acting injectable versions.

The story of monoamine oxidase inhibitors (MAOIs) also goes back to the early 1950s. In another chance discovery, doctors found that depressed patients taking a particular drug for TB gained some relief from depression. Further research led to the synthesis of yet more drugs that worked in much the same way. Although MAOIs were often effective, they had important side effects including hazardous interactions with common foods. Tricyclic antidepressants (like imipramine and amitriptyline) came onto the market around the same time and soon became the first choice for major depression, even if they too had their weaknesses.

In the 1980s, along came selective serotonin reuptake inhibitors. Fluoxetine, marketed as Prozac, became the most fêted but there are many SSRIs, as well as a related group of antidepressants called SNRIs, or selective norepinephrine reuptake inhibitors. While these drugs are also imperfect, they were the first psychotropics to be developed with a specific site of action as the target.

When it came to anxiety, barbiturates had been around since the early 1900s. They were effective as sedatives and sleeping pills, but they could depress breathing. Many people took too large a dose, either unintentionally or on purpose, and never woke up (See Chapter 6, page 129).

Serendipity struck again in 1955 when a researcher at Swiss pharmaceutical company Hoffmann-La Roche discovered the tranquillizer chlordiazepoxide, the first of a new class of drugs called benzodiazepines. By 1960, it was marketed as Librium. Diazepam followed three years later under the trade name Valium. At first, the benzodiazepines appeared safer than barbiturates and less likely to interfere with respiration or cause dependence. Doctors and patients went wild with enthusiasm. In no time, benzodiazepines were more widely prescribed than any other drugs. The 1966 hit 'Mother's Little Helper' highlights tranquillizer use among housewives, and the risks of addiction and overdose. The little yellow pills of the Rolling Stones' lyrics are thought to refer to Valium. Benzodiazepines aren't just habit-forming. Tolerance develops too, so that progressively larger doses are needed to get the same effect. Nowadays, doctors prescribe them far more reluctantly.

In an article he wrote in 1971, British psychiatrist William Sargant (1907–88) prophesied that the new drugs would eliminate mental illness by the year 2000. Today, he is remembered not just for this inaccurate prediction, but also for his antipathy towards any form of psychotherapy. Instead, he passionately endorsed physical remedies like psychosurgery, ECT, insulin shock therapy, and the deep-sleep treatment he pioneered. At St Thomas' Hospital in London, patients with depression underwent a regime of deep sleep or extreme drowsiness for up to three months during which they were often given ECT and antidepressant drugs, with or without their consent.

Sargant was not the only one who based treatments on personal conviction rather than science, but he stands out as more of a maverick that most. His role as a media psychiatrist and his alleged involvement in work on mind control for the security services added to a general distrust of his methods.

⋙⋘

In the 1960s and early 1970s, social and cultural change put patients' rights on the agenda on both sides of the Atlantic. There were calls for asylums to be opened up, and for assumptions about so-called madness to be re-evaluated.

The anti-ECT movement was particularly vocal, with many former patients, lawyers, social scientists, and psychiatrists all calling for the treatment to be abandoned. Popular media also played a part. There were few positive depictions of ECT. American author Ken Kesey (1935–2001) gave memorably negative images of the 'Shock

Shop', as he called it in his 1962 novel, *One Flew Over the Cuckoo's Nest*. 'Five cents worth of electricity through the brain,' says one of the patients in his book, 'and you are jointly administered therapy and punishment for your hostile go-to-hell behavior.'

Was ECT, and indeed all of psychiatry, really about manipulating people rather than caring for them? Many psychiatrists began to wonder whether a diagnosis of mental illness was merely a convenient label for behaviour that could not easily be managed. Perhaps what some experts called mental illness was just someone's way of coping in a mad world. According to Scottish psychiatrist R.D. Laing (Ronald David Laing, 1927–89), schizophrenia was a normal adjustment to a dysfunctional environment.

In the US, the Hungarian-American psychiatrist Thomas Szasz (1920–2012) was a leading light of the same movement, often referred to as 'anti-psychiatry'. Like Laing, however, Szasz rejected that label. In his opinion, most conditions considered to be mental illnesses were really problems in living. Unfortunately, psychiatry conflated behaviour and disease, so, instead of people controlling their own destiny, practitioners ended up controlling them.

There was some logic in this more modern view. Weren't rebellious women often diagnosed with hysteria? In the mid-nineteenth century, some doctors even believed that enslaved people who tried to flee were suffering from a condition called 'drapetomania'. As you might guess, a good whipping was said to prevent it.

Today, we are still uncertain as to what causes mental illness. A genetic element may exist in some cases, but the environment plays a large part. There's plenty of data suggesting that abuse, conflict, active combat, childhood neglect, and social isolation all raise the risk of mental ill health. Poverty does too, although the evidence is less robust.

∝

In the climate of the 1960s, ECT inevitably fell out of favour. Many of its problems were due to the unethical way in which it was sometimes used, for example under coercion, or at any rate without informed consent.

Yet ECT has enjoyed a revival since the 1980s. The procedure has been modified so as to be almost unrecognizable to that in Cerletti's day. Nowadays it's performed under anaesthesia, and with a muscle relaxant to reduce muscular contractions. Electrodes are often placed on only the right side of the head to minimize adverse effects.

There are still side effects. Most often, patients feel disorientated and dozy after the session, feelings that usually pass. There can also be muscle pain and headache after ECT. More seriously, some get antegrade amnesia, meaning that they can't remember well after the treatment. Others may develop retrograde amnesia, which involves loss of memory for events that occurred before their shock treatment. For a few, amnesia can be severe and distressing, especially if it goes back years and includes biographical memories.

According to a recent estimate, around 100,000 Americans a year receive ECT. The main reason for its current use is severe depression that fails to respond to other treatments. ECT is no longer recommended for schizophrenia, but it can be useful for bipolar disorder and mania. While the treatment still carries something of a stigma, many patients and psychiatrists – and people who are both – endorse it.

How does ECT work? In the many decades since it was developed, there has been theory after theory. Cerletti himself spent years researching this and became convinced that *l'elettroshock* made the brain release chemical mediators that restored mental health. He named these substances *acro-agonins* from the Greek words for 'extreme' and 'struggle'. He went as far as to inject patients with a preparation made from the brains of pigs who had been electroshocked. Despite his zeal, the effects were disappointing.

Nobody talks of *acro-agonins* anymore. And yet the concept of active substances within the brain looks a lot less far-fetched since the discovery of neurotransmitters. These are chemical messengers that carry signals from one nerve cell to the next target cell, which is often another nerve cell. So far, over 100 neurotransmitters have been identified. They include serotonin, glutamate, gamma-aminobutyric acid (GABA for short), dopamine, and various endorphins.

These days, after studies with brain imaging and hormone assays, we finally know a bit more about the mode of action of ECT. While it may not be the whole story, there's evidence that GABA is involved in its antidepressant effect. In some respects, you could say that Cerletti's bizarre theory foreshadowed the discovery of neurotransmitters, as well as the development of drug therapy for mental ill health. Both ECT and the drug chlorpromazine can raise levels of the hormone prolactin. This may not be significant. Then again, it may be one more piece of evidence suggesting that ECT and psychopharmacology are not so very different after all.

It would be a mistake to caricature Cerletti as a single-minded scientist bent on dishing out electric shocks to both animals and humans. He took a far wider view of mental illness and recognized that mental hospitals were not the right environment to help people. He believed that, with their huge impersonal wards, most of them offered entirely the wrong milieu. To make the neuropsychiatric clinic in Genoa less forbidding, he removed the bars from the windows, which must have seemed very progressive at the time. In 1949, Cerletti wrote in the journal *Il Ponte*, 'Is it reasonable for us to treat people who have lost their mind by making them live amongst others who have lost theirs too?' He went on to say, 'They have nothing of their own, not even their chair, no personal items of furniture, no drawers or personal effects. How can they possibly find themselves again?' The best part of a century has passed since then, and most people can agree that every patient should be treated as a person, just as Cerletti suggested.

Meanwhile, the burden of mental ill health is ever growing. In the UK, one in five adults – or about 8.6 million people – are now prescribed antidepressants, with no prospect of those numbers falling. When it comes to children aged eight to sixteen, one in five living in England has a probable mental health condition, according to an NHS report in 2023. Eating disorders in particular have risen. Increased awareness of mental disorders is healthy, but there is also a risk that common problems such as grief, stress, and distress are being medicalized. That is perilously close to the way in which troublesome behaviour was traditionally treated, especially in women. Today there's still not enough focus on the factors that lead to ill health like conflict, poverty, neglect, and social isolation. As Laing and Szasz believed, many mental disorders may really be problems in living.

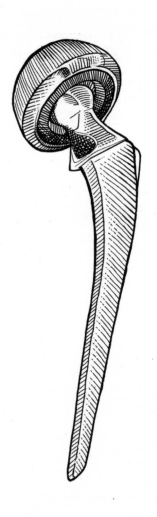

11

The Prosthetic Hip:
A Triumph of Orthopaedics

Arthritis of the hip is not new. Skeletons from ancient Britain show its presence. Even Neanderthal man had arthritis.

In osteoarthritis, the most common kind of arthritis, the smooth cartilage that covers the joint surfaces becomes worn. Without cartilage, the joint no longer moves as freely. The bone that lies beneath the cartilage hardens and eventually develops cysts and bony spurs around the joint margin. Movement is increasingly painful and limited, and life can become severely restricted. Before hip replacements, people coped by walking with a stick or limping with crutches, until their condition led to increasing immobility and confinement to the home or even to bed.

Treatment of joint disease was rudimentary for most of recorded history. Before anaesthesia and blood transfusion, the surgical possibilities were limited to how long a patient could stand the agony, or how long until they bled to death. Even for those who survived an operation, infection was a frequent killer afterwards.

For centuries, surgery developed in tandem with war. Bloody conflicts and ubiquitous firearms made limb amputation a much-needed procedure to save life. Lopping off an injured or diseased member was far quicker, easier, and surer than anything else. It was the number one solution to skeletal problems in civilian life, too. Eventually, the rising status of surgeons and the arrival of antisepsis and anaesthesia enabled the development of other limb operations.

Until well into the twentieth century, operating on bones and joints was regarded as a branch of general surgery. Today, orthopaedics is an established speciality in its own right. Even so, other doctors still mock its practitioners: 'An orthopod is as strong as an ox and almost half as intelligent.' A dip into the history of hip replacement, however, should convince anyone that so-called orthopods are, in reality, inventive and thoughtful, and many bring skills learned elsewhere to find innovative solutions.

'Orthopaedics' refers to making children straight. The term originated in 1740, when Nicolas Andry (1658–1742), a former dean of the Paris School of Medicine, coined it for the title for his book *Orthopaedia*, in Latin. Since then, the world has adopted the word. Today, however, most orthopaedic patients are adults rather than growing children. In describing the practice of orthopaedics, Andry recognized the role of muscles in moulding and stabilizing the body. Deformities, he believed, could be both prevented and cured by the right exercises. This principle still holds true. Mobilization is vital to recovery from orthopaedic surgery, and maybe even from all operations.

Hip replacement is the crowning glory of orthopaedics. It has transformed the existence of millions. Neither kidney transplants nor coronary artery bypass grafts surpass hip replacement for improving quality of life. A new hip may not add years to life, as cardiac surgery can, but it adds life to years.

It took until the twentieth century for hip replacement surgery to come into its own. First, the medical profession had to embrace the concept of limb preservation rather than amputation. In 1761, Prussian surgeon Johann Ulrich Bilguer (1720–96) was one of the first to propose limb-sparing interventions, but few medics of the time adopted them.

London surgeon Anthony White (1782–1849) is said to have carried out the first successful procedure to remodel or restore the function of a hip joint – an operation called arthroplasty. It was 1821 and his patient was a nine-year-old with TB of his hip. In times past, TB of the hip and other bones was common and affected all ages, not just the middle-aged and elderly. Hip pain and a limp are early symptoms. As destruction of cartilage and bone progress, there can be severe pain as well as deformity, leg shortening, and restricted movement. Sometimes there are also general symptoms of TB, such as night fever and weight loss. A child with TB hip did not have much of a future.

White did not replace the boy's hip, but he did remove the diseased head of the femur, in other words, the most troublesome half of the hip joint. His operation was deemed so heroic that two senior surgeons threatened to report him to the Royal College of Surgeons in London. As it turned out, the nine-year-old patient did so well that White dispatched him to call on the detractors to change their minds.

White was either constitutionally lazy or shockingly late. He often missed appointments altogether, yet he grew a large and fruitful practice. An able surgeon, his audacious operations included cutting out the bottom half of the jaw in one patient, and removing the lower end of the femur in another.

Although White usually gets the credit for the first excision arthroplasty of the hip, Liverpool doctor Henry Park (1744–1831) may have got there before him. The notes that Park made of the patients he treated are not that legible, but it seems that he attended at least one duel and many births, including that of William Gladstone in 1809, who went on to become Prime Minister. Park also wrote to a mentor about removing a hip joint to treat disease. It's not clear whether he intended new bone or fibrous tissue to fill the gap. Either way, it seems he hoped some sort of healing would, with luck, fulfil the functions of a joint. Thus began the chequered history of hip surgery, a tale of ingenuity and experimentation.

In 1826, John Rhea Barton (1794–1871) from Philadelphia performed the first osteotomy of the hip. This involved cutting the upper end of the femur between the greater and lesser trochanters in the hope of helping a man who'd lost movement in his stiffened hips. The ambidextrous Barton was a skilful surgeon and completed the osteotomy in seven minutes – just as well, since there was no anaesthetic. A few weeks later, the patient was encouraged to keep his muscles working. Three months later, he was walking with a stick. Movement had prevented bone healing post-op, and a pseudarthrosis or fake joint had formed in its place. Unfortunately, the procedure didn't bring lasting relief. The joint continued to degenerate and cause pain. Barton is also known for introducing bran dressings to treat compound fractures, in which there's an open wound near the break so that broken ends of bone may protrude through the skin. What Barton failed to appreciate was that bran makes an ideal home for bedbugs.

In 1854, another American surgeon showed a progressive approach to TB of the hip. Lewis Sayre (1820–1900) was all for removing the head of the femur and allowing nature to create a new joint of sorts. In this, he anticipated Gathorne Robert Girdlestone's signature operation (of which more later) by over seventy years. Sayre treated over seventy patients in this way, but many of them died.

Sayre also made a name for himself in his management of spinal disorders, in which he was equally progressive. He treated patients with twisted spines by suspending them from a frame by their arms. However, possibly his most startling treatment came when he saw a five-year-old boy whose legs were so severely contracted that he was unable to walk upright. Sayre considered cutting the hamstring tendons and using electricity to stimulate the muscles. Just then, a nurse piped up to warn him that the boy's 'pee-pee' should not be touched as it was very sore. Sayre immediately inspected the painful part, noted the boy's tight foreskin, and carried out a circumcision. In no time, the boy was able to stand. He allegedly walked home two weeks later. Sayre admitted that he was unsure how the remedy had worked, but he was nonetheless wholly convinced that circumcision could help musculoskeletal problems in children, and even improve behaviour and intelligence. It was Sayre who helped change circumcision from a religious and cultural practice into a medical procedure.

⤬

But back to the hip. By the mid-nineteenth century, it was clear that simply cutting out the joint might occasionally relieve pain, but what was left of the hip was unstable and let patients down. Something more was needed. American surgeon John Murray Carnochan (1817–87) was bold enough to carry out some of the most challenging operations known to date, and a few more besides. He took out an entire jaw, and removed another patient's forearm bones while saving the arm and its function. In 1840, he removed a hip joint and put wooden blocks in its place.

Others proved equally inventive. In 1860, Parisian surgeon Aristide Auguste Stanislas Verneuil (1823–95) interposed soft tissue into the resected hip, and with that he began a trend. In 1885, Louis Léopold Ollier (1830–1900) from Lyon chose to use fatty tissue instead. Ollier had a distinguished record in treating war injuries, but inserting fat into joints proved less successful. He did, however, go on to use anaesthesia, antisepsis, and X-rays in his practice, and is often considered a founder of French orthopaedics. Several other illustrious names from Lyon became interested in bone surgery around this time, though not all focused on conserving tissue. Surgeon Mathieu Jaboulay (1860–1913) successfully performed amputations through the middle of the pelvis.

The late nineteenth century was an era of daring experimentation. Eminent physician Themistocles Gluck (1853–1942) from Berlin should be fêted for creating the first ball-and-socket replacement joint. In 1891, it was a design well in advance of its time. Made from ivory, it was roughly similar in shape to a natural hip joint, and it was fixed to the bone with screws. Gluck also fashioned replacements for other joints, the possibilities being limited only by the imagination and whatever materials were to hand. To illustrate the range of his work, Gluck had a complete skeleton fitted with joint replacements that included the shoulder, elbow, wrist, knee, and ankle as well as the hip. Known as the 'skeleton of Paris', it was displayed until the Second World War before it vanished. Unfortunately, infection led to many failures of Gluck's operations. Most of his work remained unpublished because of a rift with his chief, another reason why Gluck is under-recognized today.

Czech Vitezslav Chlumsky (1867–1943) was another innovative surgeon. In 1896, he experimented with a range

of substances, interposing materials such as muscle, celluloid, silver plates, rubber struts, wax, magnesium, zinc,
glass, and decalcified bones. It was Robert Jones (1857–
1933) who tried gold, presumably mined in his native land.
Born in Wales, Jones became an orthopaedic surgeon
in Liverpool where he installed an X-ray machine only
months after the rays were discovered (see Chapter 9). He
used it to locate a bullet in a twelve-year-old boy's wrist.
These were the earliest days of X-rays and exposure took
two hours, a long time to keep still with a bullet lodged in
your hand. The image was the first X-ray to appear in a
medical journal. It marked the beginning of the close part-
nership between orthopaedics and radiography.

Around 1902, Jones had a patient whose hips had
completely seized up, with solid bone uniting the femur and
the pelvis. Jones freed the hips and managed to reconstruct
them, using gold foil to cover the femoral heads. Twenty-
one years on, the patient had good movement and very
little pain. At that point, it was the longest follow-up in
the history of hip arthroplasty. Jones is also known for his
collaboration with the British nurse Agnes Hunt (1866–
1948). Their legacy is the Robert Jones and Agnes Hunt
Orthopaedic Hospital, a specialist centre in Oswestry,
Wales. Jones saved many lives during the First World War
with his pioneering treatments and his organizational flair.
Thanks to him, orthopaedic hospitals grew across Britain.

⤸

At the beginning of the twentieth century, there was still
a long way to go before hip replacement became reality.

John Benjamin Murphy (1857–1916) from Chicago is mainly remembered as an abdominal surgeon, majoring in the gall bladder. Born in a log cabin to Irish immigrants who had fled the potato famine, he was baptized plain John Murphy, but gave himself a middle name when he noticed that everyone else had one. Murphy spotted that arthritis often caused osteophytes, or bony spurs, around the joint. He believed that chipping these away would be curative. Unfortunately, it wasn't.

Murphy and colleagues also tried inserting fascia lata into the hip joint. This meant taking some of the tough fibrous sheath – the fascia lata – from around the thigh muscles, and grafting it into the hip. Meanwhile, various other surgeons tried pig bladder. For a while this seemed a firm favourite because it stood up well to pressure within the joint. If the patient survived, so would the pig bladder inside the hip. Would rubber be even more resilient? French surgeon Pierre Delbet (1861–1957) thought it promising. He created a rubber prosthesis to replace the femoral head in 1919, but the results didn't last.

In the 1920s, Marius Nygaard Smith-Petersen (1886–1953) had a light bulb moment. Based in Boston, the Norwegian-American surgeon fashioned a glass mould to fit over the head of the femur. He had noticed that the human body tolerated glass well on a long-term basis. Operating on a patient with glass in his back, Smith-Petersen once found a glistening sac with a few drops of clear fluid, not unlike a normal joint. His plan was to encourage cartilage regeneration on both sides of his moulded glass hemisphere and then remove it later. Unfortunately, the glass shattered as it couldn't cope with the demands of walking. Smith-Petersen then tested celluloid, Pyrex, and Bakelite (which broke and caused squeaking). In 1937, his dentist suggested Vitallium, an alloy of 65 per cent cobalt, 30 per cent chromium and 5 per cent molybdenum. Recently introduced to dentistry, Vitallium resisted corrosion. Smith-Petersen and his colleagues worked on a cup arthroplasty which he affixed to some 500 hips. It was the first series of promising results for arthroplasty using a material inserted into the joint.

British surgeon Ernest William Hey-Groves (1872–1944) made a return to ivory in the 1930s. Born in India, he was a general surgeon who carried out a number of experiments in orthopaedics and bone grafting, but his ivory hip did not work out long term.

The 1930s and 1940s were still the heyday of TB, when surgeon Gathorne Robert Girdlestone (1881–1950) from Oxford set to cutting out the head of the femur in those with TB and other joint infections. Girdlestone was a man of deep religious beliefs and his passion for this operation bordered on evangelical. As he put it, 'If thine femoral head offend thee, pluck it out and cast it from thee.' His procedure removed the septic area. After this surgery, soft tissues fill the gap and take the load. However, the leg ends up shorter and rotates outwards because of the shape of the pelvis. The hip is far less stable as a result, so the person needs walking aids. Today, surgeons still sometimes use the Girdlestone operation as a salvage procedure after a failed total hip replacement.

For replacing hips, the most promising material so far was metal. Philip Wiles (1899–1967), a London surgeon who had worked with Smith-Petersen, described the UK's first total hip replacement with stainless steel components attached to the bone with screws and bolts. Unfortunately, results were disappointing. Wiles was an altruist whose ideals often led him to champion the underdog. In the 1930s, he attended wounded republicans in the Spanish Civil War and arranged medical care for the Red Army in China.

In 1940, South Carolina surgeon Austin Moore (1899–1963) took metal further when he was faced with a weighty problem in the shape of a forty-six-year-old man of about 113 kg (250 lb). A tumour at the upper end of his femur led to recurrent fractures. One solution was to amputate at the hip. The other was to make a valiant attempt at creating a bespoke hip replacement, which Moore did with fellow surgeon Harold Ray Bohlman (1893–1979) from Nebraska. The implant was 30 cm (12 in) long with a large head made of Vitallium. They attached it to the shaft of the man's femur with bolts. Moore arranged for the epic surgery to be filmed. The spectacle was bloody. The patient's recovery was equally turbulent, but he survived and became mobile once again. When he died two years later, it was from heart disease. The partial hip replacement had worked. What's more, it showed no signs of wear.

The two surgeons improved the design of their implant, and the final model had a fenestrated stem that fitted into the upper end of the femur and encouraged bone growth around it. This helped anchor it securely without bolts. The Austin Moore prosthesis, as it became known, was the first joint replacement to be widely available off the shelf. It found its way into thousands of hips all over the world. It also took pride of place on the bonnet of Moore's 1951 Chrysler Imperial.

Because of the unique arrangement of blood vessels near the head of the femur, fractures of the upper neck of the femur cannot heal on their own. They need surgical help. For many years, the Austin Moore implant was used for this purpose, although nowadays the trend is to replace the whole hip, both femoral head and pelvic cup.

In those early days, hip surgeons see-sawed between metal and other materials, and to some extent the debate continues today. Over in Paris, the Judet brothers, Jean (1905–95) and Robert (1909–80), were both prominent professors of orthopaedic surgery. They pioneered the Judet acrylic hip prosthesis in the late 1940s. Unfortunately, the acrylic made squeaking sounds. Worse, it often crumbled, but a few patients were lucky and their hips still functioned decades later. The Judet brothers also had mixed fortunes. In the 1970s they were prosecuted for tax fraud and stripped of their Légion d'honneur medals as well as their professional status. In 1981, however, they were both cleared of all charges.

For years Vitallium had the edge when it came to implant longevity. Norman Sharp was five years old when septic arthritis destroyed both hip joints and left him in pain, unable to walk. He was twenty-three when he had his first hip replacement, performed by Philip Newman (1911–95), orthopaedic surgeon and Dunkirk hero. It was December 1948, and the procedure at the Royal National Orthopaedic Hospital, London, was said to be the first of its kind in the brand-new NHS. Three weeks later, Sharp's other hip was replaced. In 2019, the *Guinness Book of Records* recognized Sharp, by then in his nineties, as owning the oldest surviving hip replacements. The Vitallium implants had served him well for over seventy years.

The early 1950s saw a flurry of activity as surgeons continued to perfect Vitallium components. By then, TB was on the decline. It is still common in the developing world, but by the mid-twentieth century in Britain the condition took up fewer resources and fewer hospital beds, leaving medics to attend to other conditions. In England, surgeons Kenneth McKee (1906–91), John Watson-Farrar (1926–99), and Peter Ring (1922–2018) all developed metal-on-metal joint implants of varying designs.

But how to secure the components to bone? Most surgeons used acrylic cement – methyl methacrylate – another favourite with dentists. Peter Ring, however, became the king of cementless hips, developing the Ring prosthesis which needed no cement. The pelvic component was fixed with metalwork. Later models had a polyethylene cup, but it turned out these were more likely to wear out than the original metal-on-metal versions.

What if a total hip implant could be made to minimize wear at the articular surfaces? Enter John Charnley (1911–82), the British surgeon who took hip replacement to another level with his concept of low-friction arthroplasty. In his stellar career, he changed the look of everything: the implant, the operating theatre, and even the surgeon.

As a junior doctor, Charnley worked at Manchester Royal Infirmary where he had his first taste of orthopaedics, a speciality still regarded as minor. When the Second World War broke out, he worked with the Royal Army Medical Corps and found an outlet for his ingenuity at the first Base Ordnance Workshop, in Abbassia, Egypt, where he designed several bits of equipment, such as a walking caliper and surgical instruments. Once back in the UK, Charnley worked at the Robert Jones and Agnes Hunt Hospital in Oswestry. Forever inquisitive, he wondered what might happen if one implanted bone both above and below the periosteum (the tissue layer that covers and nourishes bone). To find out, he convinced a junior doctor to experiment on him. The result was infection of his shin bone, which needed several operations to put right.

Returning to Manchester, Charnley worked on hip implants. Mindful of the Judet brothers' prosthesis which squeaked and failed, he researched joint friction and lubrication. Until then, most artificial hips had components of the same size as a natural femoral head and acetabulum (pelvic socket). Charnley's designs, developed with engineers, had a much smaller head (22 mm in diameter instead of 40 mm) and a smaller cup to match. This had the effect of reducing both friction and the forces acting on the implant.

Unlike a natural joint, metal-on-metal offered no lubrication so, for the socket component, he chose polytetra-fluoroethylene (PTFE), otherwise known as Fluon®, from Imperial Chemical Industries (ICI). PTFE was amazingly smooth and its surface had the inherent slipperiness of a skate on ice. Unfortunately, it was less durable than predicted and wore down within two years. Even worse, debris from it caused adverse reactions in many patients. At this point, Charnley considered giving up on hip replacement.

However, he had two great allies. Harry Craven (1928–2007) was a young fitter and turner who came to Charnley as an assistant in 1958 from the Metal Box Company. His remit was to test implant materials and make surgical tools in Charnley's attic. As Craven said in an interview, 'There was no money and no materials to make the thing with, so I used to go to a scrap yard up the road and see what they had got.'

Craven's greatest contribution was testing ultra-high molecular weight polyethylene (UHMWPE). Charnley had told him not to bother with this new plastic, but Craven went ahead anyway, making use of the boss's absence in Zurich on a travelling fellowship. Craven's testing showed that UHMWPE showed less wear in three weeks than PTFE showed in twenty-four hours. Charnley saw these results on his return from Switzerland, and he was impressed. Typically, he did a little experiment and injected his own thigh with fine particles of both PTFE and UHMWPE. PTFE triggered an adverse reaction, but the new material didn't. UHMWPE was exactly what was needed. The first operation with it went ahead at Wrightington Hospital in November 1962, using polymethyl methacrylate cement. This had already proved its worth as a cement not only in dentistry but also in neurology for refashioning skulls.

It's not enough to choose and implant a durable hip. Deep infection is a devastating side effect of joint surgery, and, despite normal precautions, about 1.5 per cent of Charnley's hip replacements became infected. The implant is a foreign body that can form a nest for bacterial growth. Once infection takes hold, it can lead to total failure of the joint. Charnley was determined to take every possible measure against it.

This is where Hugh Howorth (1919–2004) came in. An air engineer, businessman, and racing driver, Howorth worked with Charnley in devising a theatre ventilation system. With its high-efficiency particulate air filtration (HEPA), the new system also directed air flow away from the operation site to reduce the chances of contamination.

Still, Charnley realized that surgeons and theatre staff breathed out bacteria that could circumvent a mask. He therefore designed a special hood and gown. With Howorth's input, that became a helmet and a one-piece gown that fitted over the helmet. The visor covered the entire face, and a tube near the mouth and nose dealt with expired air. The Full Body Exhaust system came into use in 1970. Charnley also took to wearing two pairs of gloves while operating. But that wasn't all. He introduced an operating enclosure to fit inside the theatre. Patient and operating staff went inside it, while the anaesthetist remained outside. Dubbed the greenhouse, the enclosure had side panels that could be removed for cleaning, or perhaps when the theatre was used for surgery other than joint replacement. With all these precautions in place, the infection rate fell to 0.5 per cent.

Charnley was a skilled surgeon who could safely operate two or three times faster than his colleagues. His eye for detail was just as impressive. He turned his attention to the role of cement and realized that, rather than working as a glue, it was more of a grout, filling spaces in the bone like a jigsaw puzzle. Charnley used generous amounts of cement and applied it into every nook and cranny of the femur, so that it would hold the implant as firmly as possible.

Charnley's results were excellent. Was further improvement feasible? Some believed so. In the 1970s, French surgeon Pierre Boutin (1924–89) developed a ceramic on ceramic (CoC) bearing. However, squeaking, popping, and grinding were sometimes a problem. Sound effects do not necessarily indicate imminent failure of the implant, but they can be disconcerting.

Since Charnley, cement has again come under the spotlight. Now there are more implants that can be used without it. Today, more uncemented hip replacements are done, with cemented versions used for revision surgery, if the first hip implant fails. It's also become clear that hip components sometimes need to be tailor-made, for instance, for young patients or those from different parts of the world. In theatre, more surgeons now make use of computer assistance to help fix the implant into its optimal position.

～

Several designs for total hip replacement give excellent long-term results in terms of function and relief from the pain of arthritis – and at a cost that pleases health economists. At least, that's the case for patients over sixty-five. But arthritis tends to affect just the joint surfaces, and a more bone-sparing method might be more suitable for younger people. An artificial hip only needs to replace the layer of worn cartilage and a few millimetres of bone beneath it. So-called resurfacing arthroplasty is a technique that leaves the neck of the femur in place while the head is resurfaced with a cap. While the concept is not new, the procedure only took off in the mid-1990s.

British surgeon Derek McMinn (b. 1953) pioneered hip resurfacing and developed the Birmingham Hip Replacement, which is now the longest-serving hip implant of this type. Such implants cost more and take longer to put in, but the procedure also causes less blood loss. Unfortunately, they're not a panacea. In women, older patients, and those with smaller hips, results tend to be less certain because of bone thinning and osteoporosis. Birmingham Hip Resurfacing is best for physically active men with a hip larger than 50 mm, in whom long-term results are usually excellent.

Typically, resurfacing implants are metal–on–metal. It seems that a small number of patients develop metallosis: in other words, inflammation, pain, or allergy from metal particles that rub off the implant. If this happens, there's little alternative but to swap the implant for a conventional full total replacement.

While the hip has the longest track record of any joint replacement surgery, these days many more joints – knees, shoulders, elbows, ankles, and even fingers can be safely and effectively swapped for artificial implants. When the joint that nature handed you doesn't stay the course, surgeons can restore movement and banish pain.

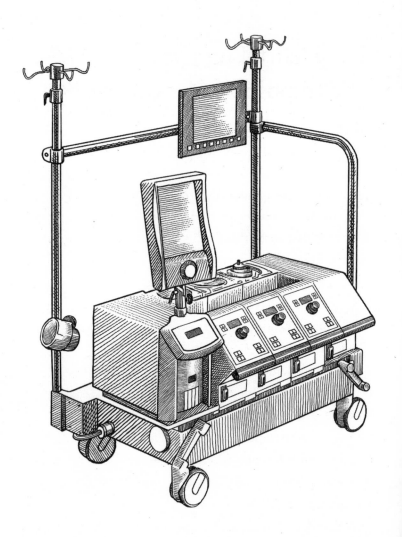

12

The Heart–Lung Machine: How the Impossible Became Possible

The heart is unique. Limbs can relax. Even the brain can rest sometimes. The heart cannot. It beats on average once a second, or nearly three billion times in a person's lifetime. Of course, lungs are vital organs too and, like the heart, their movement is obvious even to a casual observer. But there are two of them, and they hardly carry the same significance. What poet has ever pledged his lungs to his true love?

Surgery demands a still and bloodless field. But the heart is in continuous motion, pumping 5 l (1 gallon) of blood every minute. Many warned that operating on the heart was impossible. It's just as well they did. As US surgeon Clarence Walton Lillehei (1918–99) put it, 'Once they said it could not be done, it was a sufficient challenge to do it.'

All of that makes cardiac surgery one of the most sensational advances in medicine. The heart–lung machine, also known as the cardiac bypass machine, has made it possible to save the lives of those with congenital heart anomalies, rheumatic heart disease, coronary artery narrowing, and many other conditions besides. Worldwide, over a million cardiac operations are now done a year using the heart-lung machine. In most cases, the mortality rate is just 1 or 2 per cent.

Heart surgery had a shaky start. 'No surgeon who wished to preserve the respect of his colleagues would ever attempt to suture a wound of the heart.' These words are attributed to German surgeon Theodor Billroth (1829–94). Whether or not he said them at a meeting of the Vienna Medical Society in 1881 is uncertain, but it was very much the prevailing attitude. Surgery on the heart was out of the question.

That didn't deter Ludwig Rehn (1849–1930). In 1896, the German surgeon was faced with a twenty-two-year-old gardener who had been stabbed in the heart with a knife. At the time, the treatment for cardiac wounds was absolute quiet, the application of leeches, and, perhaps, if the physician felt brave, drawing off some fluid from around the heart. But the gardener was getting worse, so Rehn went in, stitching a wound measuring 1.5 cm (½ in) in the man's right ventricle. It was the world's first success-ful cardiac operation.

British surgeon Henry Souttar (1875–1964) was the first to deliberately cut into a heart. Trained initially as a mathematician and engineer, he had wide interests and an innovative mind. In 1925, fifteen-year-old Lilian from East London was desperately ill as a result of rheumatic fever. Although rare today, rheumatic fever was rife in the pre-penicillin era. Due to an immune reaction to a bacterial infection like scarlet fever or strep throat, rheumatic fever is an acute illness that attacks the heart valves and heart muscle. Rheumatic heart disease is the name given to its long-term effects on the heart. In Lilian's case, the mitral valve was critically narrow. She was also suffering from recurrent attacks of rheumatic fever and involuntary movements known as chorea. On top of this, she had asthma. Souttar proposed opening her heart through the left atrium and dilating the mitral valve. His colleagues believed it would be manslaughter.

Souttar went ahead anyway. On 6 March 1925, Lilian was put to sleep with alcohol, chloroform, and ether. There was no anaesthetist as such, just one of Souttar's fellow surgeons holding a face mask while an assistant checked on the pulse and refilled the ether vaporizer as and when. Lilian breathed on her own throughout her surgery, even though her ribs had been cut, her chest opened, and her left lung collapsed. Souttar went in through the auricular appendage and passed a finger in and out of the mitral valve a few times. He had designed a sharp instrument – a valvotome – for the occasion but decided against using it because he could now feel that the valve wasn't just rigid and tight. It leaked too (a condition called 'incompetence'), and he didn't want to make it worse. As it was, each time his finger was inside the valve, Lilian's wrist pulse disappeared.

Perhaps surprisingly, given that Souttar only tinkered with her valve, Lilian improved. But she was never wholly well and had a further attack of rheumatic fever. A stroke killed her six years later. Souttar and colleagues went on to repair further mitral valves. The results were abysmal. Of ten cases, only two survived the post-op period, and only one of these got better. Surgeons had shown that the heart could be opened, but could any good come of it? Nobody was convinced, and valve surgery came to a halt for about twenty years.

✂

A hundred years ago, rheumatic disease was one of the most common acquired heart conditions, but there were also congenital abnormalities, many of which were fatal in childhood. American surgeon Robert Gross (1905–88) was chief surgical resident at Harvard Medical School and an able operator despite only having sight in one eye. In 1938, he came up with the idea of surgically correcting a patent ductus arteriosus in a seven-year-old girl.

The ductus arteriosus is a blood vessel connecting the pulmonary artery to the aorta, so that blood bypasses the lungs. This is the norm in every baby in the womb, but the ductus arteriosus is meant to close soon after birth. If it stays patent, too much blood flows to the lungs. While a small patent ductus may not cause trouble, a sizeable one leads to fluid build-up in the lungs. In these cases, the heart has to work harder, and the baby has trouble feeding and even breathing. They may even go blue (cyanosed) from lack of oxygen. In theory, a ductus could be operated on without opening the heart itself, but it was a huge risk. Gross's boss, the chief surgeon William E.

Ladd (1880–1967), forbade him to take on this procedure. Gross waited. Once Ladd sailed off on his annual voyage to Europe, Gross operated on the girl. She survived. After successfully tying off his first patent ductus, Gross went on to operate on other congenital anomalies and he inspired a generation of surgeons.

American surgeon Dwight Harken (1910–93) was a larger-than-life military medic from Iowa. Harken arrived in England with the US military in preparation for the D-Day landings. He was thirty-four when he was appointed to manage the 160th US General Hospital, a rambling field hospital in the grounds of Stowell Park, Northleach, Gloucestershire. It bore more than a passing resemblance to a string of Nissen huts, but it contained all the equipment Harken needed.

Tall, red-haired, and somewhat temperamental, Harken turned out to be just right for the job. In the last year of the war, he busied himself removing bullets and shell fragments from the chests of 134 soldiers. In fifty-six cases, these were inside the heart. Even so, every single one of his patients survived, even Sergeant Leroy Rohrbach. An explosion at the Battle of Normandy had sent a piece of shrapnel flying into Rohrbach's chest, where it embedded in his heart. Harken had already tried twice to remove it. At the third attempt, there was a torrential haemorrhage. Harken managed to plug the wound in the heart with one finger. The operation was a success, although Harken had stitched a finger of his glove to the patient's heart.

Many eminent surgeons came to the field hospital to watch and learn during Harken's eighteen months in Britain. Once he was back in the US, word of his successes spread there, too, and led to huge interest in heart surgery. If it was possible to open the heart to remove metal and repair wounds, surely more could be feasible.

Harken went on to repair and even design replacement valves. His patient Mary Richardson made history. She survived twenty years after Harken replaced her aortic valve with a ball-in-a-cage artificial valve. At the Peter Bent Brigham Hospital, Harvard, he implanted the first pacemakers. In his obituary, the *New York Times* called him the Father of Heart Surgery.

⁓

The final years of the Second World War saw further attempts to treat congenital heart defects. In coarctation, there is a localized narrowing of the aorta, which causes increased pressure before the narrowed segment and poor blood flow beyond it. Many believe that Robert Gross was the first to repair coarctation of the aorta in 1945, though in reality Swedish surgeon Clarence Crafoord (1899–1984) had got there before him the previous year.

Gross and Crafoord succeeded, but many operations of the time failed. It didn't help that the diagnostic methods were basic, usually no more than a stethoscope and a chest X-ray. However, even with the most accurate diagnosis, many procedures were impossible. There just wasn't enough time, because the body cannot survive long without oxygen. The brain can only last four minutes before permanent damage sets in. Some doctors found another way to treat their desperately ill patients, as Helen Taussig and Alfred Blalock did in 1944.

Helen Brooke Taussig (1898–1986) was an American paediatrician at a time when there were few women in medicine. At Johns Hopkins Hospital, Baltimore, she soon found herself taken up with the care of children with congenital heart disease. Many of them had Fallot's tetralogy. Named after French pathologist Étienne-Louis Fallot (1850–1911), the four features of the complex condition are stenosis (narrowing) of the pulmonary valve and pulmonary arteries, a hole in the heart called a ventricular septal defect (VSD), a thickened right ventricle, and an enlarged aortic valve that seems to open from both ventricles because it sits atop the VSD.

Most of Taussig's little patients had profound lack of oxygen with inky blue extremities, lips, and noses. These so-called 'blue babies' were all doomed. Some of her patients with Fallot's also had a patent ductus. Those children, Taussig noticed, did better, but they deteriorated if the ductus closed on its own. She had an idea. What if a ductus, or something like it, could be created? She called on Alfred Blalock (1899–1964). Originally from Georgia, Blalock was chairman of the surgical department at Johns Hopkins. He had already done vital work on shock and blood volume replacement, which contributed to the treatment of trauma in the Second World War. Blalock also found ways to suture blood vessels together to create an anastomosis: in other words, a new junction between two tubes. In the lab, he worked with Vivien Thomas (1910–85), a young man who had come to Johns Hopkins as an unqualified assistant and did most of the animal work.

Taussig put her idea to Blalock and Thomas. Eileen Saxon was an infant so ill and so blue that she could not live outside an oxygen tent. At eleven months old, she weighed 4.3 kg (9½ lb), the same as a four-week-old baby. Was Blalock willing to operate? He replied that he was. 'You don't do a new operation on a good risk. You do a new operation on a patient who has no hope of survival without it.'

Despite the tiny size of Eileen and her arteries, Blalock, his resident William Longmire, Jr (1913–2003), and his intern Denton Cooley – of whom more later – all took part in that historic operation in November 1944. Standing right by them was Vivien Thomas, whose experience and guidance were essential to the surgery. The operation involved joining the left subclavian artery to the left pulmonary artery, in essence creating an artificial human ductus. It was something that Thomas had done in the lab, but Blalock had not.

After Eileen, other patients followed. Children from the world over were brought to Taussig's paediatric cardiac clinic, while the doctors she trained eventually migrated to all parts of the globe.

It was well known that many animal experiments, mostly on dogs, had preceded the surgery, and the anti-vivisection movement grew vocal, even threatening. Baltimore City Council held hearings. Taussig staged a parade of young patients, now healthy and active, many with their own pet dog in tow. She won the day.

That landmark operation became known as the Blalock-Taussig shunt, although the term Blalock-Taussig-Thomas would be more accurate. Thomas was an African-American with no college education. Nonetheless, as a lab assistant at Johns Hopkins, he did so much more than assist in the lab. His work was essential to the Blalock-Taussig shunt, yet he got no mention in scientific articles. Blalock was supportive, but only up to a point. Shamefully, Thomas was classified and paid as a janitor despite being an integral part of the surgical team. Eventually, he became an instructor of surgery at Johns Hopkins.

The Blalock-Taussig-Thomas shunt was a breakthrough. It gave hope to families of children with all kinds of congenital heart disease, not just Fallot's. But the operation pioneered at Johns Hopkins was only palliative. It didn't correct the underlying anomaly. That came years later, if the patient was lucky.

❦

The concept of opening tight valves arose again after Henry Souttar. Independently of one another, several surgeons, including Russell Brock (1903–80) at Guy's Hospital, London, all took up the practice of widening heart valves with one finger. The late 1940s were a busy time for those who could operate to relieve rheumatic heart disease. The surgeons all opened up heart valves blind, as Souttar had in 1925. It was the only way.

Then came a Canadian surgeon with a bright idea. If the brain was at risk when the heart was stopped, how about slowing down the metabolism of the body before stopping the heart? Toronto surgeon Wilfred Gordon Bigelow (1913–2005) had treated frostbite while serving in the Royal Canadian Army Medical Corps. Once the Second World War was over, he began researching hypothermia. Bigelow found that a body temperature of about 30°C (86°F) allowed the circulation to be stopped for ten minutes. This was long enough for a quick procedure on the heart. However, he also discovered that too steep a drop in temperature led to cardiac arrest, so it was vital to get it right. There were various possible methods of cooling a patient, but the most popular was surface cooling, either with a special blanket or by immersion in a bath of iced water. Bigelow's work also led, in 1950, to another innovation: the electronic pacemaker. As it turned out, he needed one himself a few years later.

Bigelow's colleagues might have been sceptical of hypothermia, but other surgeons were enthusiastic. Thomas Holmes Sellors (1902–87) adopted hypothermia to close atrial septal defects (ASDs), an ASD being a hole in the heart between the two atria. He operated with a lot of ice and his trademark composure. His results put Harefield Hospital, Middlesex, on the map, and surgeons from all over the world flocked to watch him at work. Holmes Sellors also carried out the first direct operation to relieve a narrowed pulmonary valve. That day, he had planned a Blalock-Taussig procedure, but the patient's lungs were too adherent to allow this. Borrowing a tendon knife from a nearby orthopaedic theatre at Harefield, he calmly cut into the pulmonary valve instead. The patient was alive and well years later.

Hypothermia enabled the very first successful open-heart operation in September 1952. It was at the University of Minnesota and the surgeon was Floyd John Lewis (1916–93). Five-year-old Nancy had an ASD. Her operation began with immersion in iced water in a drinking trough, of the type more often seen on a farm. It took two hours and ten minutes to lower her rectal temperature to 28°C (82.4°F). The surgical team, which included Walton Lillehei, then opened her chest and shut off the blood flow to her heart. Lewis only had ten minutes in which to operate. Fortunately, he closed Nancy's ASD in just five and a half. Once done, a bath of hot water at 45°C (113°F) brought her core temperature up to 36°C (96.8°F). With cooling down and heating up, it was a lengthy procedure, but, for the first time ever, surgeons had successfully operated on an open human heart in a bloodless field. Eighteen months later, Lewis reported on a series of eleven ASD closures using this method. Eight of the patients survived.

More than many surgeons, Lewis was a man of myth and legend. Always innovative, he was a general surgeon as well as a physiologist and a proficient mathematician who foresaw the computer age. It was perhaps surprising that he retired suddenly at the age of sixty. He died in retirement in California, some believe of sepsis, but those who knew him say boredom finished him off.

Induced hypothermia had immense benefits at the time and is still used today in heart surgery, alongside other methods. But it could not do the job when an operation was longer and more complex. Here's where John and Mary Gibbon came in. John Heysham Gibbon was a research fellow in surgery at Massachusetts General Hospital. The inspiration for his life's work came in October 1931 in the shape of a plump fifty-three-year-old woman. Two weeks after having her gall bladder removed, she became acutely unwell with a large clot on the lung – a pulmonary embolus. Removing the embolus surgically was not an option, according to Edward Churchill (1895–1972), the surgeon in charge. The procedure had never been done in the USA and was very rarely successful anywhere else in the world. All that could be done for the woman was to keep an eye on her condition. That was the young John Gibbon's task. He sat up all night checking her vital signs and watched her get worse. She might have had a chance, he thought, if only it were possible somehow to remove the blue blood from her swollen veins, take out the carbon dioxide, add oxygen, and then return it to her circulation. But, of course, that was impossible. In the morning, Churchill decided to operate as a last resort. Although he took out the embolus in minutes, the woman died.

As for Gibbon's notion of removing blue blood and returning oxygenated blood to the body, it was a madcap idea. His father, also a surgeon, tried to persuade him to pursue something more practical than this pipe-dream.

Churchill seriously doubted it could be done, but he offered Gibbon a research fellowship to explore his epic plan all the same. He even hired Gibbon's wife.

From 1934 onwards, Gibbon and his wife, Mary Hopkinson Gibbon, spent time at Harvard devising a cardio-pulmonary bypass machine, or heart-lung machine. Mary was an educated woman who was already involved in scientific research, which was how she had met John. Together, their aim was to take over the work of the heart and lungs completely during surgery while keeping the rest of the body oxygenated and alive.

This machine needed four basic components: a pump to keep blood circulating, an oxygenator to add oxygen, a reservoir for venous blood, and a temperature regulator for the blood while it was outside the body. A Harvard engineer assisted the Gibbons, and the team used whatever materials were available. The tubing had to be latex rubber, while the connectors and cannulas were glass or metal. The gas-exchange surface of the oxygenator was the most challenging element to formulate. They decided on a rotating cylinder into the top of which blood went in. A film of blood ran down the inside surface of the metal cylinder, allowing it to take in oxygen and release carbon dioxide. To prevent blood from clotting, Gibbon used the anticoagulant heparin, a drug that had not long been discovered. In creating their machine, they had to consider damage to blood cells and possible allergic reactions to the materials. It also had to have removable parts for sterilizing between patients.

They began with animal experiments and published their early results in 1937, when they had managed to keep cats alive for four hours with the help of a basic machine. But many obstacles cropped up along the way. Finding machine parts was one. Major problems with the oxygenator included foaming and haemolysis (rupture of red blood cells). There was also the danger of air embolism. Bubbles of air or axygen can be fatal, so the entire machine, tubing included, had to be filled with blood to ensure no air got in.

The Gibbons worked on their cardio-pulmonary bypass device for over a decade, apart from the Second World War when John was a military surgeon in South East Asia. In the early 1950s, the couple invented a more effective machine, with help from IBM. By 1953, the machine was ready. It's often said that the Gibbons' first human patient was a college freshman. In fact, it was a fifteen-month-old girl who was already very unwell. Her condition was thought to be due to a large ASD but, once she was on the operating table, Gibbon found no defect. The child got worse and died without coming round from her anaesthetic.

Three months later, the second patient was eighteen-year-old Cecelia Bavolek, a freshman at Wilkes University, Pennsylvania. Gibbon operated on her ASD on 6 May 1953 at Thomas Jefferson University Hospital in Philadelphia. Total heart bypass time was forty-five minutes. Mary Gibbon was the perfusionist: in other words, the expert looking after the machine.

That operation was so successful that Cecelia Bavolek lived for at least fifty years after it. But the next five patients died. Gibbon abandoned the use of his machine and went to work on liver disease, most likely with his father's advice ringing in his ears. All the same, the survival of that one teenage patient inspired others. It showed it could be done. Gibbon did not know it at the time, but this was the dawn of surgery using bypass to take over from the heart and lungs. It was also the dawn of the new role of clinical perfusionist.

In Minnesota, meanwhile, Walton Lillehei came up with a different way of doing things. He operated on children's hearts using cross-circulation, in which one of the parents does the work of the child's heart and lungs during surgery.

His first patient in 1954 was Gregory Glidden, a thirteen-month-old with a VSD. The father had the same blood group, so he lay on another operating table next to Gregory's. A tube in Mr Glidden's femoral artery in the thigh took oxygen-rich blood to a pump that sent the blood to Gregory's aorta. Another tube took blood from one of Gregory's main veins into Mr Glidden's femoral vein for his circulation to oxygenate. Gregory's heart was still beating, but it was bloodless as Lillehei stitched up the VSD. The operation took seventeen minutes. Although Gregory survived his surgery, he died of pneumonia a few days later.

Lillehei used cross-circulation on many more occasions. Medical reactions were mixed. Some thought the technique was immoral because it put the donor at risk.

The popular press, on the other hand, was in rapture, especially when one five-year-old girl was on her tricycle seven weeks after open-heart surgery. 'A New Heart for Pamela' became front page news, never mind that it was a repaired heart rather than a new one. Publicity had benefits, not least for the blood bank. Each operation needed about 7 l (15 pints) of blood, and local residents soon flocked to become donors and help save young lives.

In some ways, cross-circulation was like a pregnancy. Also like a pregnancy, it had, as Lillehei admitted, a potential mortality rate of 200 per cent. Lillehei went on to carry out many more operations in this way, mainly on VSDs, though he also corrected Fallot's tetralogy. His results were impressive and few donors suffered, although one developed a stroke from air embolism. It was the first series of successful open-heart operations, albeit without a heart-lung machine.

But cross-circulation wasn't always feasible, so specialists put their efforts into improving the heart-lung machine. Surgeon John W. Kirklin (1917–2004) and his team at the Mayo Clinic, New York, took up where Gibbon had left off. As a student, Kirklin had been inspired by Robert Gross. Once Kirklin graduated, he and his colleagues filled notebook after notebook with their plans to fix hearts, if only they could get inside them.

After a few refinements to the pump and the oxygenator, Kirklin repaired a sizeable VSD on a five-year-old girl in 1955. She went home ten days later. However, his next few patients did less well. Of the eight in Kirklin's first series, half died. On the other hand, children with VSDs rarely lived beyond the age of six, so doing nothing was a death sentence. Kirklin continued to operate, and the outcomes improved. He went on to be one of the leading heart surgeons.

In the mid-twentieth century, two main US centres of excellence for cardiac surgery emerged – the Mayo Clinic and the University of Minnesota. Soon after the Mayo Clinic results were published, Lillehei at Minnesota gave up on cross-circulation and began using the heart–lung machine. Surgeon Richard DeWall (1926–2016) dedicated himself to improving the machine further. To tackle the problem of emboli from gas bubbles, DeWall came up with an oxygenator that had silicon antifoam and special polyethylene tubing. Over a period of two years, 350 open-heart operations took place at the University of Minnesota with the Lillehei-DeWall bubble oxygenator. Thus began a golden era of cardiac surgery.

Perhaps needless to say, patients would never have got as far as the operating table without cardiologists, physiologists, pathologists, and, of course, engineers to maintain the machinery. Inside theatre, perfusionists, anaesthetists, and nursing staff were essential members of the team. Anaesthetists had to relearn their entire way of working. For a start, a patient on cardio-pulmonary bypass can't breathe in an anaesthetic gas. It has to be given via the machine. The usual ways of monitoring the patient by checking their vital signs don't work either, because there's no pulse when a roller pump is in action.

The heart–lung machine enabled surgeons to go where they had not ventured before, but it also caused problems. Blood was in contact with non-biological materials, and they weren't compatible. The machine changed plasma proteins and activated blood cells. This had two main unwanted effects: inflammation and coagulation.

The oxygenator element continued to be a bugbear. Bubble-type oxygenators were liable to create gas and other emboli. Fat and fibrin (a large protein involved in clotting) often found their way into the brain. They were probably the cause of so-called 'pump madness', one name for the mild impairment that some had after surgery. Since then, refinements to the system have included oxygenators that use a membrane instead. Keeping operating time to a minimum is also key to reducing the risks.

⚬

The demand for valve surgery dwindled as rheumatic fever declined, but a newer challenge took centre stage. Coronary artery disease, due to narrowed arteries around the heart, became more commonplace in the second half of the twentieth century.

In 1951, Canadian surgeon Arthur Vineberg (1903–88) had an idea. He rerouted the internal mammary artery and buried it within the wall of the left ventricle to increase blood flow to the heart. Fortunately, the internal mammary artery travels down the inside of the ribcage, so it's not far away. As a bonus, it is expendable as well as less liable to blockage than the coronary arteries. Over 10,000 Vineberg operations were done, and many patients with angina benefited. But, at the time, there was no way of proving that implanting the internal mammary actually led to greater blood flow to heart muscle. As a result, many of Vineberg's peers were lukewarm about his procedure.

A much-needed way of visualizing the arteries to the heart soon arrived. It happened by accident in 1958. American paediatric cardiologist F. Mason Sones (1918–85) was using an X-ray contrast fluid to study the left ventricle when he mistakenly injected it into the patient's coronary circulation. At the time, this was thought to be highly dangerous. Terrified, Sones thought he'd killed his patient. But he hadn't. He'd unwittingly invented coronary angiography. This new investigation made it possible to delineate the coronary arteries accurately and pinpoint any blockages in them. It was finally possible to show the effects of the Vineberg operation. The proviso, however, was that one had to wait months for the full effect on the blood vessels to show up.

In 1960, a new operation arrived on the scene. German-born surgeon Robert H. Goetz (1910–2000) was the first to perform successful coronary bypass surgery when he took a section of the internal mammary artery and joined it directly to the right coronary artery on the far side of the narrowed section. His patient was a thirty-eight-year-old New York taxi driver with crippling angina. After the operation, he lived symptom-free for a year.

Coronary artery bypass surgery was to be one of the most significant advances of the century. But you wouldn't have guessed it from the way Goetz's colleagues reacted. They deemed the procedure experimental and appointed another surgeon in his place. Goetz never carried out a second operation.

It was years before the operation gained the approval of fellow medics. Also known as CABG (pronounced 'cabbage'), coronary artery bypass grafting is now one of the most common surgeries. As powerful as the treatment is, however, it's worth remembering that it only bypasses a blockage. It doesn't halt the progress of heart disease in that patient.

⚒

The 1960s were also the era of valve replacement. In 1960, American surgeon Dwight Harken was one of the first to implant an artificial valve. It was quite a feat to design a prosthesis to take the place of the aortic or mitral valve. The even greater challenge was ensuring it was compatible with human tissue and didn't trigger clotting or haemolysis. In time, two main types of valve developed: mechanical valves (like the ball-and-cage) and biological valves, which are either from human cadavers or from other species like the pig.

Centres for cardiac surgery flourished, among them Baylor College of Medicine, Houston, Texas, where Michael DeBakey (1908–2008) and Denton Cooley (1920–2016) plied their trade. There was also Stanford University in California where Norman Shumway (1923–2006) and Richard Lower (1929–2008) collaborated in the 1950s and 1960s on research that led to heart transplantation.

On 3 December 1967, South African surgeon Christiaan Barnard (1922–2001) stole the show with the world's first heart transplant. His audacious operation at Groote Schuur Hospital, Cape Town, relied heavily on Shumway and Lower's work in the USA, which he had studied in depth. But Barnard got there first. That and his glamorous persona captivated the world. His patient Louis Washkansky died eighteen days after surgery. Less than two weeks later, Barnard transplanted the heart of a young mixed-race man into the chest of Philip Blaiberg, a retired white dentist. This time, the patient survived and led an active life for more than eighteen months. Although the transplant had racist overtones to many, in fact Barnard was against apartheid. He later transplanted a white woman's heart into a black man.

It was no time before other surgeons, including Lower and Shumway, also transplanted hearts. Those early transplants led to a reappraisal of death and the acceptance of the concept of brain death. Immunosuppression was another advance that prevented rejection of the donor heart and led to better outcomes. Before long, transplant programmes almost covered the world.

A shortage of donors soon became painfully obvious. Transplants could therefore not be done for everyone who might benefit. Could a heart-lung machine be miniaturized and designed for extended use for ambulatory patients? That was the concept behind the artificial heart. It was also the impetus for ventricular-assist devices, which do exactly as their name suggests.

It takes a particular kind of person to be a cardiac surgeon: painstaking yet bold, with near endless reserves of energy, confidence, and perseverance, and of course with proverbial nerves of steel. These characteristics do not always make for easy relationships. The feud between DeBakey and Cooley ran for about forty years, making it the longest in the history of surgery. The elder of the two, Michael DeBakey was born in Louisiana to Lebanese parents with the surname Dabaghi. He met doctors at his father's drugstore and learned to sew from his mother, so perhaps it was natural that he would become a surgeon. As a young doctor, DeBakey used his wife's sewing machine to run up the first graft made of Dacron to repair arteries. He had nylon in mind, but the department store had none left. DeBakey also went on to design a knitting machine for producing grafts. However, DeBakey was not just a trailblazer in synthetic grafts for the aorta and other blood vessels. He was also one of the first to carry out coronary artery bypass surgery.

Denton Cooley was cut from a different cloth. A native Texan, he worked with Blalock at Johns Hopkins and Brock at the Royal Brompton in London before returning to the US in 1950 to work with DeBakey at Baylor College of Medicine and Methodist Hospital in Houston. At that point, DeBakey was the best-known surgeon in the world, and Baylor one of the most prestigious institutions. In 1952, DeBakey and Cooley successfully repaired an abdominal aortic aneurysm, the first Americans to do so.

In 1956, the duo adopted the improved DeWall-Lillehei heart-lung machine and went on to carry out nearly a hundred open-heart operations to repair septal defects and other congenital heart anomalies. DeBakey liked to analyze clinical data, bringing his painstaking approach to auditing as well as to operating.

DeBakey also pioneered the development of an artificial heart. In 1966, he became one of the first surgeons to use an external pump successfully. This was a left ventricular-assist device (or LVAD). The patient was a thirty-seven-year-old who'd been on the heart-lung machine but couldn't manage without it towards the end of the operation. Now, with the LVAD in place, the heart really could rest. And it did. Remarkably, this patient later had the device removed and was able to go home.

The falling out between DeBakey and Cooley took place in 1969 over a piece of plastic and Dacron weighing barely 220 g (8 oz). The artificial heart had been engineered in DeBakey's lab at Baylor. By this time, Cooley had relocated to St Luke's Hospital nearby. That was near enough for Cooley's purposes. Without approval from DeBakey or Baylor, he acquired an artificial heart from his former colleague's lab and used it for his own patient. Unfortunately, the patient only lived for two and a half days. DeBakey was furious. He himself had not yet used a total artificial heart, for the simple reason that solid evidence was still lacking.

DeBakey called Cooley's use of the heart a theft, a betrayal, unethical, and childish. Cooley justified his actions with his view that the patient was in desperate need. Besides, the Russians had gotten there first with the Sputnik, and he didn't want them to win again.

The American College of Surgeons censured Cooley, and the fallout led to Cooley's resignation. DeBakey continued doing surgery until he was ninety, by which time he had carried out an estimated 60,000 operations and trained several thousand surgeons. As for the dispute, something like a public reconciliation finally took place in October 2007, when DeBakey was ninety-nine and Cooley was eighty-seven.

Cooley was a gifted surgeon. He was also aware of his own talent. When a trial lawyer once asked him if he was the best heart surgeon in the world, Cooley agreed that he was. The lawyer suggested that might be rather immodest. Perhaps so, Cooley conceded. 'But remember I'm under oath.'

Transplants have become increasingly successful. However, there's an eternal shortage of donor hearts. Perhaps the best-known artificial heart was the Jarvik 7. Engineered by American innovator Robert Jarvik (b. 1946), it was successfully implanted in 1982 at the University of Utah. In the last few decades, the Jarvik 2000 ventricular-assist device has been useful for patients with advanced heart failure who might be awaiting a transplant. The Jarvik 2000 is a titanium device the size of a large thumb. Once implanted into the left ventricle and connected to its external battery pack, it provides a continuous pulseless flow.

Other developments include operations on the beating heart. As groundbreaking as the heart–lung machine was, it still has drawbacks. A CABG is actually a procedure on the surface on the heart rather than within it, so many surgeons now choose to operate without it when they can. The main difficulty when the heart is beating is finding ways to stabilize the arteries during the intricate surgery.

There's also minimally invasive heart surgery. This took off in the 1990s and means that the chest doesn't have to be opened from stem to stern. Nowadays, the aortic valve can even be replaced without opening the chest at all. Transcatheter aortic valve replacement (TAVR) is now done in units throughout the world.

In 1998, French surgeon Alain Carpentier (b. 1933) brought robotics into the arena of cardiac surgery when he carried out the first mitral valve repair using the DaVinci robot. He has also designed valves, and has earned the title of the Father of Modern Mitral Valve Repair.

While some of the latest procedures may sound simpler than operations using cardiac bypass, they would not have been possible without initial work on the heart-lung machine. Extracorporeal membrane oxygenation (ECMO) wouldn't exist either. Inspired by the heart-lung machine, ECMO is a treatment for saving the lives of critically ill patients whose lungs temporarily don't function. This can happen with a severe infection, including some cases of Covid-19. With ECMO, blood is pumped from one tube into the membrane oxygenator and then passed back to the patient's bloodstream through a second tube.

So the machine effectively takes over from the lungs. The procedure was developed in the USA and the first successful treatment of an adult was in 1971. Treatment takes place in a few specialized units, some of which can treat young children.

Bilroth and his contemporaries would be amazed. The reality today is the ability not just to operate on the heart, but to replace it. You could say that all conditions of the heart are potentially treatable. Alas, the causes of heart disease are still with us and have yet to be tackled.

Timeline

10,000 BCE Evidence of trepanation, one of the first
surgical procedures

460 BCE Birth of Hippocrates of Kos (*c.*460 BCE–*c.* 370
BCE), the Greek father of medicine, marking a more
scientific study of medicine

129 CE Birth of Galen of Pergamon (129–216 CE), Greek
physician, surgeon, and philosopher

980 CE Birth of Avicenna (980–1037 CE), Muslim
philosopher and physician

1348 Onset of the Black Death in Europe, a pandemic
of bubonic plague (ends 1353)

1510 Birth of French barber-surgeon Ambroise Paré
(*c.*1510–90)

1514 Birth of Andreas Vesalius (1514–64), deemed the
world's greatest anatomist

1628 William Harvey publishes *Exercitatio Anatomica
de Motu Cordis et Sanguinis in Animalibus* (An
Anatomical Disputation of the Movement of the
Heart and Blood in Animals), known as de *De Motu
Cordis*, showing how blood flows around the body

1642 English Civil War begins (ends 1651)

1656 British architect and inventor Christopher Wren
(1632–1723) experiments with intravenous
injections into dogs, and later into one human

1665 Onset of the Great Plague of London, the worst outbreak of plague in England (ends 1666)

1665 British scientist Robert Hooke (1635–1703) discovers cells under the microscope

1676 Dutch microscopist Antonie van Leeuwenhoek (1632–1723) reports the sighting of 'animalcules' under his microscope

1697 Birth of William Smellie (1697–1763), Scottish apothecary who wrote *Treatise on the Theory and Practice of Midwifery* and is often dubbed the Father of Midwifery

1738 Irish midwife Mary Donally (dates unknown) performs the first caesarean in which the mother survives

1753 Scottish physician James Lind (1716–94) publishes his *Treatise of the Scurvy* on the preventing of scurvy with citrus fruits

1768 Birth of Astley Paston Cooper (1768–1841), English surgeon and anatomist

1775 American War of Independence begins (ends 1783)

1789 French Revolution begins (ends 1799)

1794 Birth of Robert Liston (1794–1847), Scottish surgeon and inventor of the Liston knife

1796 British physician Edward Jenner (1749–1823) said to develop vaccination for smallpox, the first vaccine against any disease

1799 British chemist Humphry Davy (1778–1829) discovers the anaesthetic properties of nitrous oxide

1803 Napoleonic Wars begin between France and multiple countries (end 1815)

1811 Birth of James Young Simpson (1811–70), Scottish obstetrician, forceps designer, and pioneer of anaesthesia for labour

1816 French physician René Laennec (1781–1826) invents the stethoscope

1821 London surgeon Anthony White (1782–1849) is said to carry out the first successful procedure to restore the function of the hip joint

1842 American pharmacist and surgeon Crawford Long (1815–78) uses ether as an anaesthetic for the first time, but does not publish his work

1844 American dentist Horace Wells (1815–48) uses nitrous oxide as an anaesthetic

1846 American dentist William Morton (1819–68) is credited with showing that inhaled ether works as an anaesthetic

1847 British doctor John Snow (1813–58) invents an ether inhaler and becomes the first doctor to specialize in anaesthetics

1847 Hungarian physician Ignaz Semmelweis (1818–65) discovers how to prevent the transmission of puerperal fever

1849 Elizabeth Blackwell (1821–1910) becomes the first woman to gain a medical degree in the US

1853 Frenchman Charles Gabriel Pravaz (1791–1853) develops the first hypodermic syringe, using it in sheep

1853 Scottish physician Alexander Wood (1817–84) develops the first plunger-operated hypodermic syringe and uses it on human patients

1853 John Snow dispenses chloroform to Queen Victoria for the birth of Prince Leopold

1857 French photographer Abel Niépce de Saint-Victor (1805–70) discovers that uranium salts give off radioactivity

1861 Beginning of US Civil War (ends 1865)

1861 French biologist Louis Pasteur (1822–95) publishes his germ theory of disease

1865 Louis Pasteur patents pasteurization

1865 Elizabeth Garrett Anderson (1836–1917) becomes the first woman to qualify as a doctor in Britain

1865 French neurologist Pierre Paul Broca (1824–80) discovers the brain's speech centre

1867 British surgeon Joseph Lister (1827–1912) publishes his treatise *On the Antiseptic Principle in the Practice of Surgery* and first uses his carbolic spray

1877 British anaesthetist Joseph Thomas Clover (1825–82) designs the first inhaler that properly regulates the amount of ether inhaled

1882 German microbiologist Robert Koch (1843–1910) formulates his criteria for establishing that a microorganism causes a particular disease. He also isolates and cultures the tubercle (TB) bacillus

1884 British surgeon Rickman Godlee (1849–1925) performs the first operation to remove a brain tumour

1889 American surgeon William Stewart Halsted (1852–
1922) introduces the use of rubber gloves to the
operating theatre

1891 German surgeon Themistocles Gluck (1853–1942)
designs the first ball-and-socket replacement hip
joint

1894 French-German instrument-maker Hermann
Wülfing-Lüer (1836–1910) develops the first
all-glass hypodermic syringe

1895 French surgeon Eugène-Louis Doyen (1859–1916)
introduces the first electrically powered bone saw

1895 Wilhelm Conrad Roentgen (1845–1923) discovers
X-rays

1896 French physicist Antoine Henri Becquerel (1852–
1908) is credited with discovering radioactivity

1896 German surgeon Ludwig Rehn (1849–1930)
performs the first successful heart operation when
he stitches the heart of a man who had been
stabbed

1896 Austrian neurologist Sigmund Freud (1856–1939)
founds psychoanalysis

1897 German-Polish surgeon Johann Mikulicz-Radecki
(1850–1905) designs the first surgical face mask

1898 French physicist Pierre Curie (1859–1906) and
French-Polish physicist Marie Curie (1867–1934)
discover polonium and radium

1901 Austrian immunologist Karl Landsteiner (1868–
1943) and colleagues discover three ABO blood
groups

1908 Norwegian obstetrician Christian Kjelland (1871–1941) designs forceps that can rotate a baby's head

1911 Birth of Swedish professor Tage Malmström (1911–95), who popularized ventouse delivery in the 1950s

1911 Birth of John Charnley (1911–82), British surgeon who designed low-friction hip implants

1914 First World War begins (ends 1918)

1918 Beginning of the Great Influenza epidemic, dubbed 'Spanish flu', due to the H1N1 influenza A virus (ends 1920)

1922 Insulin first used to treat diabetes

1925 British surgeon Henry Souttar (1875–1964) attempts the first heart valve operation

1928 British microbiologist Alexander Fleming (1881–1955) discovers penicillin

1931 German physicist Ernst Ruska (1906–88) devises the first electron microscope

1933 British general practitioner Grantly Dick Read (1890–1959) publishes *Natural Childbirth*, his first book on gentle labour. It is followed in 1942 by *Childbirth without Fear*

1934 Hungarian neuroscientist László Meduna (1896–1964) first uses injections of camphor in oil to trigger convulsions in patients with schizophrenia

1936 Portuguese neurologist António Egas Moniz (1874–1955) performs the first prefrontal leucotomy in humans

1937 Karl Landsteiner (1868–1943) and Alexander Wiener (1907–76) discover the Rhesus blood group system

1938 American surgeon Robert Gross (1905–88) performs the first operation to correct congenital heart disease

1938 Italian neuropsychiatrist Ugo Cerletti (1877–1963) designs the first machine for delivering electric shock treatment (ECT)

1939 Second World War begins (ends 1945)

1944 Swedish surgeon Clarence Crafoord (1899–1984) repairs the first coarctation of the aorta

1944 The first Blalock-Taussig-Thomas operation for 'blue babies'

1947 American orthopaedic surgeon and inventor Homer Hartman Stryker (1894–1980) patents the oscillating bone saw

1950 Canadian surgeon Wilfred Gordon Bigelow (1913–2005) begins to develop hypothermia to lower metabolism and allow open-heart surgery. He also develops the electronic pacemaker

1950 Korean War begins when North Korea invades South Korea (ends 1953)

1952 American surgeon John Lewis (1916–93), using hypothermia, performs the first successful open-heart operation

1953 American John Heysham Gibbon (1903–73) performs the first operation using the heart-lung machine that he and his wife, Mary Hopkinson Gibbon (1903–86), developed

1958 American paediatric cardiologist F. Mason Sones (1918–85) accidentally invents coronary angiography

1960 Chlordiazepoxide (Librium) is first marketed

1960 German-American surgeon Robert H. Goetz (1910–2000) carries out the first coronary artery bypass graft

1966 Lebanese-American surgeon Michael DeBakey (1908–2008) implants an external heart pump

1967 South African surgeon Christiaan Barnard (1922–2001) performs the first human heart transplant

1971 British engineer Godfrey Hounsfield (1919–2004) performs the first CT scan on a patient

1973 American physicist Michael E. Phelps (b. 1939) creates the PET scanner

1978 British physicist Peter Mansfield (1933–2017) tests the first full body MRI prototype

1978 Birth of Louise Brown, the first test-tube baby

1988 Launch of the antidepressant fluoxetine (Prozac)

1991 British surgeon Derek McMinn (b. 1953) pioneers hip resurfacing procedures

1998 French surgeon Alain Carpentier (b. 1933) carries out the first robotic mitral valve repair

Acknowledgements

Only a dozen objects grace this book, but many more than twelve people helped produce it. The idea grew out of conversations with Tris Payne, so the very least I can do is thank him first. Special thanks also go to my exceptional agent Sam Brace, also at Peters Fraser + Dunlop.

The team at Quarto has been brilliant, especially Richard Green, Phoebe Bath, Michael Brunström, and the publicity and marketing squad, not forgetting the cover designer, who used my favourite colour.

I owe a huge debt to colleagues and staff at Newnham College, Cambridge, for their enthusiasm, advice, and technical support. Many thanks to fellow Newnham Fellows Jane MacDougall and Helen Taylor for their medical expertise, as well as to Peter Jaye of St Thomas's Hospital, London. Any and all errors are, of course, mine.

I'm grateful for use of the world-leading resources of the Hunterian Museum at the Royal College of Surgeons, London, and the Whipple Museum, Cambridge. With seventeen floors of books, the University Library, Cambridge, has been a peerless source for research, and it is so well organized that I didn't get lost in over 130 miles of shelves.

On a more personal note, my colleagues and friends of the Sanctuary writing group have provided invaluable support and sustenance. I also want to thank my family, especially my husband, Jeremy, to whom I owe a huge debt of gratitude for his consistent encouragement, not to mention about 200 suppers.

Finally, I'd like to acknowledge people most of whose names I've long forgotten. Over the years, patients and medical colleagues taught me that medicine isn't just about knowing how to wield an instrument. One must also learn when to use it, and when to hold back and use a technique sometimes called MICLO (masterly inactivity and cat-like observation).

Carol Cooper

Picture credits

p8 The Trephine: Science History Images/Alamy Stock Photo; *p30* The Bone Saw: Album/Alamy Stock Photo; *p48* The Mask: Bob Venables; *p70* The Microscope: Igor Golovniov/Universal Images Group/Getty Images; *p92* The Stethoscope: Channarong Pherngjanda/Alamy Stock Vector; *p116* The Ether Inhaler: Universal History Archive/Universal Images Group/Getty Images; *p138* The Hypodermic Needle and the Syringe: Channarong Pherngjanda/Alamy Stock Vector; *p162* Obstetric Forceps: Quagga Media/Alamy Stock Photo; *p186* The X-Ray Machine: Bob Venables; *p214* The ECT Machine: Bob Venables; *p236* The Prosthetic Hip: Bob Venables; *p256* The Heart-Lung Machine: Bob Venables.

Index

3M 54, 110

Abbott, Gilbert 121
accouchement forcé 178–80
accoucheurs 166–7, 168
Adler, Alfred 227
air tractor 173–4
Alcmaeon of Croton 23–4
Alexander, Albert 85
Alexandra of Denmark 127
Alzheimer, Alois 217
ambulance volante 37
amputation 30–47, 122,
    127, 135, 238
anaesthesia 13, 19, 27, 41,
    117–37, 173, 175, 179,
    238, 273
    *see also individual types of
    anaesthetic*
Anderson, Elizabeth
    Garrett 5
Andry, Nicolas 238
angioplasty 212
animal research 4, 20, 265
anthrax bacilli 82
antibiotics 83–5, 91
antidepressants 229, 234–5
antimicrobials 91
antisepsis 65, 80
antiseptic surgery 58–9,
    79–81
Argou, Jacquette Guichard
    114
Aristotle 76
arthritis 237, 254
arthroplasty 239, 244–6
asepsis 65, 80, 81
asthma 106, 107
asylums 223–4, 225, 230
atrial septal defect (ASD)
    266–7, 270
Auenbrugger, Leopold 101

auscultation 101
Austin Moore prosthesis 248
Avicenna 163, 169
awake craniotomy 27

Babcock & Wilcox 195
bacteria 73, 83–5, 88–9,
    90–1
bacteriology 81–3
barber-surgeons 32–6, 47,
    143
barbiturates 129, 229
Barnard, Christiaan 276–7
Barnes, Robert 174
Barton, John Rhea 240–1
battlefield injuries 32, 33–5,
    37, 42–4
Bavolek, Cecilia 270–1
BCG (*bacille Calmette-
    Guérin*) 83
Beatrice, Princess 124
Becquerel, Antoine Henri
    190, 191, 192
Becton, Maxwell W. 152
Becton-Dickinson 152–3
Béhier, Jules 147
Beijerinck, Martinus 87–8
Bennett, Alexander Hughes
    18
benzodiazepines 229–30
Bernays, Martha 136
Bichat, Xavier 100
Bier, August Karl 136–7
Bigelow, Wilfred Gordon
    266
Bilguer, Johann Ulrich 239
Billroth, Theodor 258, 282
Bini, Lucio 217, 218–19
Bird, Golding 108
Birmingham Hip
    Resurfacing 254–5
birth 163–85

Black, Joseph 118
Black Death 50–1
Blaiberg, Philip 277
Blalock, Alfred 263–4, 278
Blalock-Taussig-Thomas
    shunt 265
Bloch, Felix 207–8
blood 150–1, 156
    blood extraction 143
    bloodletting 143–4
    blood tests 159–60
    blood transfusions 59,
        151, 155–7
blood pressure 67–8, 108
Bloodgood, Joseph Colt 61
Bohlman, Harold Ray
    247–8
bone saw 30–47
Boutin, Pierre 253
Boyle, Robert 75
brain 12, 14–16, 25–6
    brain surgery 18–23,
        26–7, 221–3
    ECT and mental illness
        215–35
    epilepsy 17–18, 216
Brandt, Kristian 175
Broca, Paul 14, 16–17, 219
Broca's aphasia 16
Brock, Russell 265
Broglie, Louis de 89
Burke, William 39

CABG (coronary artery
    bypass) grafting 275–6,
    280–1
caesarean section
    (C-section) 183–5
Caius, John 150
Calmette, Albert 83
Cammann, George Phillip
    109

carbolic 59, 80–1
Carnochan, John Murray 242
Carpentier, Alain 281
Cassen, Benedict 205
cells 75
Cerletti, Ugo 217–19, 232, 233, 234
Chain, Ernst Boris 84–5
Chamberlen, Hugh the Elder 165–6
Chamberlen family 163–5, 169, 170
Charette, François de 96
Charles I 164
Charles IX 34, 36
Charlotte, Princess 177–8
Charnley, John 250–3
Charrière, Cutler Joseph-Frédéric-Benoît 42
Charrière bone saw 42
Chateaubriand, Céleste 104
Chateaubriand, François-René de 104
chloroform (CHCl₃) 3, 19, 79, 118, 120, 123, 124–6, 128–9, 133, 173
chlorpromazine 228, 234
Chlumsky, Vitezslav 243–4
cholera 82, 125
Churchill, Edward Delos 268–9
Churchill, Frederick 41–2
circumcision 242
cirrhosis 106
Clément, Jules (Julien) 166–7
Clostridium difficile 68, 112
Clover, Joseph 126–7, 134
eoarctation 262
coats, white 66–8
coca 135–6
cocaine 135–7
Code of Hammurabi 32
Colton, Gardner Quincy 120–1
Comins, Nicholas 109
Commodus 12

computerized axial tomography (CAT scanning) 2, 197–9, 212
Cooley, Denton 264, 276, 278–80
Cooper, Astley Paston 5, 38, 39
Cormack, Allan MacLeod 199
coronary angiography 275
coronary artery disease 274
Corvisart, Jean-Nicolas 96–7, 101
Covid-19 49, 50, 54, 55, 57, 88, 281
cowpox 86–7, 88
Cox, Margaret 145
Crafoord, Clarence 262
Craven, Harry 251
Croft, Sir Richard 177–8
Crookes tube 187–9
curare 132–3
Curie, Marie 191–3
Curie, Pierre 191–3
Cushing, Harvey 20–2, 26
Cushing's syndrome 21

Damadian, Raymond Vahan 210–11
Davy, Humphry 2, 118
de Hevesy, George 201
De Quincey, Thomas 158
DeBakey, Michael 276, 278–80
deep-sleep treatment 230
Delaunay, Paul-Marie 98
Delbet, Pierre 245
Denman, Thomas 168–9, 177
dental work 63, 120, 121, 134
depression 228–9, 233
DeWall, Richard 273
DeWall-Lillehei heart-lung machine 278
diabetes 157–8
Dickinson, Fairleigh S. 152
dissection 24–5, 38–9, 100, 150

Donald, Ian 195–6
Donally, Mary 184
Doyen, Eugène-Louis 45
Drebell, Cornelis 72
Drew, Charles R. 156–7
drug abuse 158–9
ductus arteriosus 260–1, 263

ECMO (extracorporeal membrane oxygenation) 281–2
ECT (electroconvulsive treatment) machines 215–35
Edison, Thomas 2–3
Edward VII 127
egophony 104–5
Ehrlich, Paul 84, 91
electron microscopes 89–90
Elsholtz, Johann Sigismund 141–2
epidemics 73–4, 86
   see also Black Death; Covid-19, etc
epidural anaesthetic 137
epilepsy 17–18, 216
Erasistratus 24
ether 41–2, 117–37
eye protection 54–5

facemasks 49–58, 69
Fallot, Étienne-Louis 263
Fallot's tetralogy 263, 265, 272
Faraday, Michael 118
FDG (2-fluro-2-deoxy-D-glucose) 203
Ferrier, David 20
fillet 169
Fleming, Alexander 84
Florey, Howard Walter 84–5
Flügge, Carl 52
fluorinated hydrocarbons 133
fluoroscopy 194–5
FONAR 211
Forbes, John 103
forceps, obstetric 163–85

Fowler, Joanna Sigfred 202, 203
Fracastorius, Hieronymus 73–4
François II 34
Franklin, Benjamin 218
Freeman, Walter Jackson II 221–3
Freud, Sigmund 136, 226–7
Full Body Exhaust system 252–3
Fulton, John Farquhar 200, 219–20
functional MRI (fMRI) 210

GABA 233–4
Gage, Phineas P. 15–16
Galen 11–12, 24, 25, 34, 97–8, 139
Galilei, Galileo 71–2
gall bladder 59
Galvani, Luigi 217
gangrene 79–80
gas and air 137
Geer, Letitia Mumford 152–3
George IV 38, 177, 178
germ theory 64, 76–7, 78–9, 82
Gibbon, John Heysham 268–71
Gibbon, Mary Hopkinson 268, 269–71
Gigli, Leonardo 44
Gigli saw 44, 47
Gillies, Harold 128–9
Girdlestone, Gathorne Robert 241, 246
Gladstone, William 240
Glidden, Gregory 271
gloves, surgical 58–64, 69
Gluck, Themistocles 243
Godlee, Rickman J. 19, 20
Goetz, Robert H. 275–6
Golgi, Camillo 25–6
Goodyear, Charles 58
Goodyear Rubber Company 60

gowns, surgical 64–5, 69
Greener, Hannah 124
Griffith, Harold 133
Gross, Robert 260–1, 262, 272
Guérin, Jean-Marie 83
Guillotin, Joseph-Ignace 95
gut microbiome 90–1

Hall-Edwards, John 189–90
halothane 133
Halsted, William Stewart 59–61, 136
Hampton, Caroline 60
handwashing 61, 78
Hare, William 39
Harken, Dwight 261–2, 276
Harlow, John Martyn 15–16
Harvey, William 98, 150–1
heart 105–6, 113–14, 151
heart-lung machine 257–81
Henderson, Mr 18–19, 20
Henri II 34
Henri III 34
Henri IV 51
Henrietta Maria, Queen 164
hepatitis 95, 133, 154, 159
Herophilus 24
Hey-Groves, Ernest William 246
Hildebrandt, August 136–7
hip prosthesis 237–55
Hippocrates 10–11, 32, 50, 68, 99, 101, 139, 143, 163
HIV (human immunodeficiency virus) 55, 88, 159
Hoffman-La Roche 229
Holmes, Oliver Wendell 2
Holmes Sellors, Thomas 266–7
homunculus 21
Hooke, Robert 74–5
Hoskin, Cyril Henry 28
Hounsfield, Godfrey 197–8, 199
Howorth, Hugh 252

humours 97–8, 143
Hunt, Agnes 244, 250
Hunter, Charles 149–50
Hunter, John 135, 171
Hunter, William 171
hygiene 77–80, 141–2
HYPAK syringe 153
hypodermic syringes and needles 129, 134, 139–61
hypothermia 266–8

Ingvar, David H. 202
Innocent VIII, Pope 140, 155
Innocent XII, Pope 72
insulin 157–8, 159–60, 218, 219, 223
intravenous (IV) 140, 141
Ireland, John 158
Ivanovsky, Dmitri 87–8

Jaboulay, Mathieu 243
Jack the Ripper 40
Jackson, Charles 121–2
Jackson, John Hughlings 17–18
Jacksonian epilepsy 17–18
jalap resin 141
James, Henry 18
James I, King 150
Jarvik, Robert 280
Jarvik 7 280
Jenner, Edward 85, 86–7, 135
Jex-Blake, Sophia 174
Joliot-Curie, Frédéric 201
Joliot-Curie, Irène 193, 201
Jones, Robert 244, 250
Joslin, Elliott Proctor 157
Judet, Jean and Robert 248, 250
Jung, Carl 227

K1 auto-disable syringe 159
Kennedy, Rosemary 222
Kesey, Ken 231
Keynes, Geoffrey 155
Keynes, John Maynard 6

Kirklin, John W. 272–3
Kjelland, Christian 175
Kjelland forceps 175
Koch, Robert 81–2
Koch's postulates 81
Koller, Carl 136

Ladd, William E. 261
Laennec, Mériadec 114
Laennec, René Théophile
  Hyacinthe 93–7, 100–1,
  102–7, 112, 114–15
Laing, Ronald David 231,
  235
Landsteiner, Karl 156
Larrey, Dominique Jean
  37–8, 135
laser cutting 45–6
Lassen, Niels A. 202
lateral pubiotomy 44
latex gloves 62–3
Lauterbur, Paul 208, 210,
  211
Lavoisier, Antoine 119, 133
Leared, Arthur 109
Leborgne, Louis Victor 16
leeches 143–4
Leeuwenhoek, Antonie
  Philips van 72–3, 74–5
Lennon, John 28
Leonardo da Vinci 49
Leopold, Prince 124
Levret, André 167
Lewis, Floyd John 267–8
Lilian 258–60
Lillehei, C. Walton 257, 267,
  271–2, 273
Lillehei-DeWall bubble
  oxygenator 273
Lima, Pedro Almeida 220–1
limb surgery 30–47
Lister, Joseph 19, 59, 64, 65,
  79–81
Liston, Robert 39–42, 122,
  172
Liston knife 40, 42, 47
Littmann, David 110
lobotomy 221–3
local anaesthetic 134–7

Long, Crawford 122
Longmire, William Jr 264
Lorme, Charles de 50–2
Lorme, Jean de 51
Louis XIII 51
Louis XIV 51, 166, 167
Lower, Richard 276, 277
Lüer, Jeanne Amélie 152
Lüer syringe 151–2
Luer-tipped syringe 154–5

McCartney, Paul 28
MacEwen, William 65
McKee, Kenneth 249
McMinn, Derek 254
MacVicar, John 196
Magill, Ivan Whiteside
  128–9
magnetic resonance
  imaging (MRI) 199,
  205–13
Major, Johann Daniel 141
Malmström, Tage 183
Malpighi, Marcello 72
Man, Albon 2
man-midwives 165, 168,
  170, 178
Manchurian plague 53
Mansfield, Peter 208–9,
  210, 211
Marcus Aurelius 12
Marie, Pierre 217
Mask-Induced Exhaustion
  Syndrome (MIES) 56
masks 49–58, 69
Maudsley, Henry 5, 224–5
Mauriceau, François 166
al-Mawsili, Ammar 142–3
medical imaging 187–213
Medici, Queen Catherine
  de 164
Meduna, Ladislas (László)
  216
mental illness 215–35
Mesmer, Franz 118
mesmerism 117–18
Metrazol 216–17, 219
miasma 50, 78, 79, 125
micro-reciprocating saws 45

Microneedle 161
microscopes 25, 26, 71–91
midwives 167–8, 169–72,
  177, 180
Mikulicz-Radecki, Johann
  52, 61
military medicine 33–5, 37,
  42–4, 103, 127–30, 135,
  156–7, 189, 193, 218,
  238, 261–2
Minié, Claude-Étienne 43
Minie ball 43
Mitchell, Silas Weir 227–8
Moniz, António Caetano de
  Abreu Freire Egas 220–1
monoamine oxidase
  inhibitors (MAOIs) 228
Monoject 153–4
Moore, Austin 247–8
Moore, James 135
morphine 136, 142, 145,
  149, 158–9, 179, 180
Morton, William 120,
  121–2, 131, 173
Moss, Angelo 200
Mountespan, Madame de
  (Françoise-Athénaïs
  de Rochechouart-
  Mortemart) 166–7
Moynihan, Berkeley
  George Andrew 61–2
MRSA (methicillin-resistant
  Staphylococcus aureus)
  68–9, 91, 112
Murdoch, Colin 154
Murphy, John Benjamin
  245
muscle relaxants 132–3

N95 respirator mask 53–4,
  57
Nancy 267
Napoleon III 127
needles, hypodermic 129,
  134, 139–61
Nelms, Sarah 87
Nembutal 129
nerve compression 135, 136
nervous system 26

INDEX

Neuber, Gustav Adolf 65
neurosurgery 8–14
neurotransmitters 233–4
Neville, William 174–5
Neville Barnes forceps 174
Newman, Philip 249
Nightingale, Florence 127,
  145
nitrile gloves 63, 64
nitrous oxide (N_2O) 118–19,
  120, 121, 127, 133, 137
Novo Nordisk 158
nuclear magnetic resonance
  imaging (NMRI) 208–9,
  210
Nufer, Jakob 183–4

obstetric forceps 163–85
Ollier, Louis Léopold 242–3
O'Neill, Alice 184
opiates 158–9
opium 117, 142
orthopaedics 237–55
Osborne, William 168
osteoarthritis 237
osteotomy 240–1
Our Bodies, Ourselves 182

pacemakers 266
pain 117–37
Pan 140
Paré, Ambroise 33–6, 178
Park, Henry 240
Pascal, Blaise 140
Pascal's law 140–1
Pasteur, Louis 52, 64, 75–7,
  78–9, 81, 85–6
pasteurization 76
PCR (polymerase chain
  reaction) 90
pectoriloquy 113
Peel, Sir Robert 127
Penfield, Wilder Graves 21–2
penicillin 84–5, 89
Penject 158
Pentothal 129–31
percussion 101–2
personal protection
  equipment 49–69

petoriloquy 105
phantom limb pain 34–5
Phelps, Michael E. 204
Pinard, Adolphe 111
Pinard horn 111
Pinel, Philippe 96
plague 50–1, 53, 83, 141
plasma 156–7, 274
Pliny the Elder 49
polio 88, 153
Porter, John B. 128
positron emission
  tomography (PET)
  199–205, 212
power saws 45
Prausnitz, Mark 160–1
Pravaz, Charles Gabriel
  146–7, 148
prefrontal leucotomy
  219–21
Priestley, Joseph 118
propofol 130–1
psychiatry 215, 227, 231
PTFE
  (polytetrafluoroethylene)
  251–2
Ptolemies 24
puerperal fever 77–9
pulmonary embolism
  106–7
Purcell, Edward Mills 207–8

Rabi, Isidor Isaac 206–7
rabies 86, 88
radiotherapy 193–4
Raleigh, Sir Walter 132
Ramon y Cajal, Santiago
  26
Rampa, Lobsang 28
Read, Grantly Dick 180–1
Rehn, Ludwig 258
rest cure 227–8
resurfacing arthroplasty
  254–5
rheumatic fever 259–60,
  274
Richardson, Mary 262
Ring, Peter 249
Riva Rocci, Scipione 108

robotics 46–7, 69, 281
Rochechouart-Mortemart,
  Françoise-Athénaïs de
  166–7
Roentgen, Wilhelm Conrad
  187–9, 190
Rohrbach, Leroy 261–2
Royal College of Surgeons
  5, 38, 47, 240
Ruska, Ernst 89
Rutherford, Ernest 201
Rynd, Francis 144–6, 160

Saint-Victor, Abel Niépce
  de 190–1
Sakel, Manfred 218
Salk, Jonas 153
Sargant, William 230
Satterlee, Richard
  Sherwood 43–4
Satterlee bone saw 43–4, 47
saws, bone 30–47
Sawyer, William 2
Saxon, Eileen 264
Sayre, Lewis 241–2
scanning electron
  microscope (SEM) 90
scanning transmission
  electron microscope
  (STEM) 90
schizophrenia 216, 218, 223,
  226, 228, 231, 233
Schmidt, Gerhard Carl 191
scintiscanner 205
scrubs 69
sedatives 129
seizures 216–19
selective serotonin reuptake
  inhibitors (SSRIs) 229
Semmelweis, Ignaz Philipp
  77–9
sepsis 83–4, 85
Sharp, Norman 248–9
Shumway, Norman 276,
  277
Simpson, James Young
  122–3, 147, 171–4, 183
Simpson's forceps 173, 175
Sims, John 178

single photon emission
computed tomography
(SPECT) 205, 210
smallpox 86–7, 88
Smellie, William 170–1, 176
Smith-Petersen, Marius
Nygaard 245–6, 247
Snow, John 3, 123–5, 126,
127
Sokoloff, Louis 202
Sones, F. Mason 275
Souttar, Henry 258–60,
265–6
sphygmomanometer 108
Sprague-Rappaport
stethoscope 110–11
Squibb 132
Squier, Ephraim George
13–14
Staël, Madame de 104
Staphylococcus aureus 68–9
stethoscope 92–115
straitjackets 225–6
Stryker, Homer Hartman
45
succussion 101
Suckling, Charles 133
Swan, Joseph 2
syringes, hypodermic 129,
134, 139–61
Syrinx 139–40
Szasz, Thomas 231, 235

Tabern, Donalee 129
talc 62
Taussig, Helen Brooke 263,
264, 265
TB (tuberculosis) 82–3, 84,
100, 106, 114, 189, 194,
228, 239, 240, 246, 249
temporal lobe epilepsy
(TLE) 17–18
therapeutic embolization
212
Thomas, Vivien 264, 265
Thomson, Joseph John
(J.J.) 89
Tiemann, George and
Co 44

transcatheter aortic valve
replacement (TAVR)
281
transfusions 142, 155–7
transmission electron
microscope (TEM)
89–90
transorbital lobotomy
222–3
trepanation 8–14, 27–9
tricyclic antidepressants 228
trypanophobia 160
tuberculin 82
Turnbull, Sara Little 54
twilight sleep 179–80

UHMWPE (ultra-high
molecular weight
polyethylene) 251–2
ultrasound 195–7

vaccines 83, 85–7, 153, 160
van Leeuwenhoek's disease
74
variolation 86
vectis 169
ventouse 174, 183, 185
ventricular septal defect
(VSD) 263, 271, 272–3
Verneuil, Aristide Auguste
Stanislas 242
Vesalius 25
Victoria, Queen 3, 103,
124–5, 127, 178
Vineberg, Arthur 274–5
viruses 85–9, 90–1
Vitallium 246, 247, 248–9
vivisection 264–5
Volta, Alessandro 217
Voltaire 3
Volwiler, Ernest Henry 129

Warren, John 121
Washkansky, Louis 277
waste, medical 64
Watson-Farrar, John 249
Watts, James Winston 221–2
Weiner, Albert 154
Wells, Horace 120

Wendell Holmes, Oliver Sr
131–2
Wernicke, Carl 17, 219
Wernicke's aphasia 17
White, Anthony 239–40
white coat hypertension
67–8
white coats 66–8
Wiener, Alexander Solomon
156
Wiles, Philip 247
Willis, Dr Thomas 99–100
Wolf, Alfred Peter (Al)
202–3
Wood, Alexander 147–9,
150, 151
Wren, Christopher 140–1
Wrigley, Arthur Joseph
175–7
Wrigley's forceps 175–7
Wu Lien-teh 53
Wülfing-Lüer, Hermann
152

X-ray machines 2, 21,
187–213, 244

Yale Luer-Lok Syringe 153

Zentino, Señora 13